R

es Myths

"Sometin ⟨...⟩ ⟨...⟩abetes, as Riva Greenberg's inspiring book shows you! This myth-busting power-house is a 'must-read' for anyone with diabetes. The stories about other people with diabetes (herself included) that she weaves into the book are further proof that what we don't know about diabetes—or what we erroneously think we know—can oftentimes be more damaging than diabetes itself."

—SHERI COLBERG, PhD, Exercise physiologist and author of
*50 Secrets of the Longest Living People with Diabetes, The 7 Step
Diabetes Fitness Plan,* and *Diabetic Athlete's Handbook*

"An excellent resource for people who have diabetes and for those who love them. Reassuring, informative and easy to read. Debunks the myths that make diabetes harder to manage and more difficult to live with."

—RICHARD R. RUBIN, PhD, Professor, Medicine and Pediatrics,
The Johns Hopkins University School of Medicine,
Past President, American Diabetes Association

"I met Riva Greenberg a few years ago at a health fair where she was teaching other patients how to live successfully with diabetes. Now Riva puts the 'truths' about diabetes in your hands—where every pa-tient and medical professional needs it to be! She communicates vital information from top diabetes specialists across the entire spectrum of diabetes care as only a well-learned patient can—simply, empatheti-cally, with wisdom and knowing. Whether you have diabetes or treat those who do, this book may shatter what you believe—and *that's* the difference between surviving with diabetes and living a long, healthy life with diabetes."

—DONNA RICE, MBA, BSN, RN, CDE, Past President,
American Association of Diabetes Educators

"Having watched my daughter grow up with type 1 diabetes, first as a two-year-old toddler newly diagnosed to a senior in college completing her BSN, I have come to realize, as have many, that living well with diabetes is 90% information and 10% insulin. As a family, we learned how to live life well with type 1 diabetes, and along the way we encountered and overcame many of the myths that Riva Greenberg helps to dispel in this book. Early in her book, Riva reminds us that "Your diabetes education never ends." Nothing could be more important to take home than that pearl, for today's "truths" can become tomorrow's myths, and the truth after all is what sets us free—to live well with diabetes."

—JEFF HITCHCOCK, Founder of the online
community Children with Diabetes

"A comprehensive and encouraging guide to diabetes, with many helpful tips. Good for those who are new to diabetes and their families and caretakers, and for those who are tired of diabetes 24/7, and need an upbeat refresher course."

—MARSHA SHYER, NY Chapter Juvenile Diabetes
Research Foundation Board of Directors

"Having been diagnosed with diabetes 34 years ago I have heard every kind of sordid, discouraging, and hopeless message out there. The biggest lesson I've learned is that my health is up to me-I am in charge—and I cannot/will not give that responsibility to anyone else. As I transitioned to insulin after years of oral medication, I kept hearing that I had failed, that my life was ending. How helpful this book is for all of us who need to know the truth, not the fiction, of diabetes!"

—CAROLYN CRUMPLER, Diabetes Patient Mentor

"I've learned a lot about diabetes since I was first diagnosed in 1978 and today I speak to groups about better managing their diabetes. Riva Greenberg's book is an exceptional aid: She combines true-life stories with a wealth of information firmly based on medical research, and by replacing myths and fears with sound advice you will achieve better control. I learned some new things and my spirits were raised by her positive message that controlling our diabetes can give us a much better chance of leading a life with few limitations."

—BOB KOLENKOW, physicist and former
associate professor at MIT

50 Diabetes Myths That Can Ruin Your Life

50 Diabetes Myths
That Can Ruin Your Life

AND THE

50 Diabetes Truths
That Can Save It

RIVA GREENBERG

Da Capo
LIFE
LONG

A Member of the Perseus Books Group

Designed by Brent Wilcox
Set in 11.75 point Adobe Garamond by the Perseus Books Group

Library of Congress Cataloging-in-Publication Data
Greenberg, Riva.
    50 diabetes myths that can ruin your life : and the 50 diabetes truths that can save it / Riva Greenberg — 1st ed.
        p.   cm.
    Includes bibliographical references.
    ISBN 978-0-7382-1320-0 (alk. paper)
    1. Diabetes—Popular works.   2. Diabetes—Miscellanea.   I. Title.
II. Title: Fifty diabetes myths that can ruin your life.
    RC660.4.G736 2009
    616.4'62—dc22

                                                                          2009006472

First Da Capo Press edition 2009

Published by Da Capo Press
A Member of the Perseus Books Group
www.dacapopress.com

Da Capo Press books are available at special discounts for bulk purchases in the U.S. by corporations, institutions, and other organizations. For more information, please contact the Special Markets Department at the Perseus Books Group, 2300 Chestnut Street, Suite 200, Philadelphia, PA, 19103, or call (800) 810-4145, ext. 5000, or e-mail special.markets@perseusbooks.com.

10 9 8 7 6 5 4 3 2 1

To my fellow diabetes travelers
who are finding their way
to live with grace and boldness.
And to all our loved ones and
medical professionals who help us do so.

Contents

Medical Myths

Food Myths

Body Fitness Myths

Psych Myths

Practical & Practices Myths

Contributing Experts

Gerald Bernstein, Director, Diabetes Management Program, Friedman Diabetes Institute, Beth Israel Medical Center, New York. Vice President, Medical Affairs, Generex Biotechnology

Betty Brackenridge, MS, RD, CDE, Director of Professional Training, Diabetes Management & Training Centers, Phoenix, Arizona, Co-author of *Diabetes Myths, Misconceptions and Big Fat Lies!*

Robert M. Eber, DDS, MS, Diplomate, American Board of Periodontology, Clinical Professor and Associate Chair, Periodontics and Oral Medicine, School of Dentistry, University of Michigan

Megrette Fletcher, MEd, RD, CDE, LD, Executive Director, The Center for Mindful Eating

Martha Funnell, Clinical Nurse Specialist, CDE, and Adjunct Lecturer in the University of Michigan School of Nursing, and Research Investigator, Department of Medical Education, University of Michigan Medical School

Lois Jovanovič, MD, CEO and Chief Scientific Officer at The Sansum Diabetes Research Institute, Adjunct Professor of Bimolecular Science and Engineering at The University of California–Santa Barbara, and Clinical Professor of Medicine at The University of Southern California–Keck School of Medicine

Francine Ratner Kaufman, MD, Distinguished Professor of Pediatrics and Communications at Keck School of Medicine and the Annenberg School of Communications of the University of Southern California, and Head of the Center for Diabetes, Endocrinology and Metabolism at Children's Hospital Los Angeles. Past President of the American Diabetes Association and author of *Diabesity: The Obesity-Diabetes Epidemic That Threatens America—And What We Must Do to Stop It.*

Maudene Nelson, CDE and RD at the Institute of Human Nutrition at Columbia University

Ben Ortolaza, American Diabetes Association Specialist, Quality Assurance

William Polonsky, PhD, CDE, Psychologist, CDE, and Associate Clinical Professor in Psychiatry at the University of California, San Diego. Founder and CEO of the Behavioral Diabetes Institute. Author of *Diabetes Burnout* and co-author of *The Secrets of Living and Loving with Diabetes.*

Wendy Satin-Rapaport, Licensed Clinical Psychologist and Social Worker, adjunct faculty at the University of Miami Medical School, Diabetes Research Institute, author of *When Diabetes Hits Home.*

Birgitta I. Rice, MS, RPh, CHES, researcher, clinician, and educator at the Epidemiology Clinical Research Center, School of Public Health, University of Minnesota, Minneapolis, MN

Jean Betschart Roemer, MSN, MN, CPNP, CDE, Department of Endocrinology, Diabetes and Metabolism at Children's Hospital of Pittsburgh.

Janis Roszler, RD, CDE, LD/N, 2008–2009 Diabetes Educator of the Year (AADE). Host of dTalk Radio on dLife.com; author of *Diabetes on Your Own Terms*, co-author of *Sex & Diabetes*, and columnist of "Dear Janis" in *Diabetes Positive!* magazine.

Betsy Rustad-Snell, BS, RN, CDE, CPT

Lynda Schultz Sardeson, MSA, RN, CDE, Diabetes Nurse Specialist, Elkhart General Hospital, Elkhart, IN. Past President of the Northern Indiana Association of Diabetes Educators

Joe Solowiejczyk, RN, MSW, CDE, Manager, Diabetes Counseling & Training, Global Strategic Affairs, LifeScan, Inc., a Johnson & Johnson company

Kathy Spain, RN, BSN, CDE, CPT, Member of Juvenile Diabetes Research Foundation's Research Lay Review Committee and author of *Kids, Insulin Pumps and You . . . A Parent's Guide to Insulin Pump Therapy for Kids; The Diabetes Answerbook; and The Diabetes Explorer Series.*

Richard S. Surwit, PhD, ABPP, FAClinP, Professor, Chief, Division of Medical Psychology and Vice Chairman for Research Department of Psychiatry and Behavioral Sciences, Duke University Medical Center

Susan Weiner, RD, MS, CDE, CDN, Contributing Medical Producer for dLife: For your diabetes Life!

Delaine M. Wright, MS, RCEP, CDE, ACSM, and Director of Fit4D.com

Introduction

The day I heard that "diabetes is not the leading cause of blindness, kidney disease, or losing a limb," my life abruptly changed. Ever since my diagnosis thirty-two years earlier, I had lived with the fear that one of these diabetes complications would inevitably be my fate. Hearing these words, I froze in bewilderment while letting out an audible sigh of relief. These words would change my diabetes management and my life.

It was Dr. William Polonsky, diabetes psychologist and founder of the Behavioral Diabetes Institute, who uttered these fourteen words in his "Coping with Diabetes" workshop. My astonishment was mirrored in the faces of all those around me. How could it be that what we'd heard our entire diabetes lives wasn't true? Then Dr. Polonsky said, "*Poorly controlled diabetes* is the leading cause of these outcomes." In that moment I recognized the absolute power of learning a truth and the debilitating power of believing a myth. My long years of fear shifted to hope: hope that if I managed my diabetes well, facing major complications might not be my fate after all.

The following year I attended another of Dr. Polonsky's workshops. It was for people who had "gotten off track" with their diabetes management. I was there to do research because, after interviewing more than one hundred people who have diabetes, I wanted to better understand why some people are more diligent in their diabetes management than others. I learned of several reasons why people give up: They have inadequate information and/or no emotional support; they don't think their efforts make a difference; they're focused on the work of diabetes rather than on the rewards of that work; and they believe that they have to manage diabetes perfectly—a falsehood I once suffered from—and therefore feel defeated by any sort of setback. Talking with Dr. Susan Guzman, also a clinical psychologist at the Behavioral Diabetes Institute, I learned that maintaining perfect blood sugars is both unnecessary and impossible (and the effort of trying to be perfect in your diabetes management is likely to drive you insane!).

Separating myth from truth has changed the way I live with diabetes. For one thing, I live with a much more positive outlook, having learned that complications can be the exception rather than the rule if you "eat healthy," get regular physical activity, take your medicine, manage your stress, and see your doctor regularly. Second, I stay well informed about new discoveries and innovations on the horizon, and being "tuned in" has brought me a renewed sense of excitement and hopefulness. And third, I view my diabetes management as a source of pride. I respect how hard I work at it and how well I'm doing, and I see my "mistakes" as learning opportunities. But this is far from where I started.

Diagnosed with type 1 diabetes at the age of eighteen, I was put in the hospital for four days. My doctor, trying to "scare me straight," described in detail the many diabetes complications that he was convinced were in my future; indeed, the fear of one complication, blindness, came to bed with me nightly for the first several years and, thereafter, on intermittent evenings. My first dozen years of having diabetes, I lived the way most patients do: fairly uneducated and oblivious to the consequences of my actions. My commitment to my health grew slowly, over time, as I developed some minor complications from high blood sugars, then realized the vital importance of managing my blood sugar, and designed a treatment program that enabled me to do so. My resolve to manage my diabetes became steadfast and super-sized when, at forty-eight, I got married and suddenly there was someone else to whom my health was important.

Today, I am highly informed about diabetes. I speak to fellow patients across the country about forming healthful habits and finding a personal reason to commit themselves to their care, and I have spoken with dozens of experts in the field for this book. I continue to conduct interviews—collecting people's stories of how diabetes has affected them—and I am researching how positive emotions such as pride, appreciation, and forgiveness help us better sustain self-care behaviors. I also teach people that it is possible to live an exceptional life not *despite* having diabetes but *because* of it.

The day Dr. Polonsky changed my life I realized that dispelling myths puts the power of the truth into our hands, where it needs to be. Unfortunately, most patients are treated by general practitioners who are not current on the latest standards in diabetes care. Often these doctors don't have adequate time to teach patients how to manage diabetes nor are they trained to help patients with behavioral changes. So I have brought the "truths"—what you need to know in every aspect of diabetes care—to you with the help of top diabetes specialists. My work as a patient-expert (a fancy way of saying that I live with diabetes, have learned an awful lot about it, and manage it pretty successfully on the whole) has placed me amid this most generous network of diabetes professionals who give their time, knowledge, and passion to improve their patients' lives every day. My sincere hope is that this book will give you the truths you need to live your exceptional life—one that's healthy, happy, long, and fulfilling.

Note: You can find definitions of many terms and conditions referred to in this book in the glossary on page 289.

Common Myths

Eating sweets causes diabetes.

TRUTH: *Actually*, it doesn't—at least not in the way you think. Diabetes is caused by a genetic predisposition and lifestyle factors, or by an autoimmune reaction. However, in the case of type 2 diabetes, eating excessive amounts of sugar may *influence* whether or not the genes for diabetes get triggered.

Talking to groups of people with diabetes, I realize how many people still believe this myth. They're sure they got diabetes because they ate a lot of pie and ice cream as a kid or last month. In fact, while checking into my hotel in Sioux Falls, South Dakota to address a group of diabetes patients the next morning, I noticed a platter of home-baked chocolate chip cookies at the reception desk. As I eyed the cookies, debating with myself whether to indulge, the woman who was checking me in picked up a cookie and, with a wink and a smile, said, "I probably shouldn't eat this. My mother has type 2 diabetes and this may just seal my fate." Yes, she may get diabetes if she consumes too many calories and becomes overweight, but not because those calories are coming from sugar.

Diabetes mellitus is the formal name for what's commonly called diabetes—a group of metabolic disorders all characterized by abnormally high blood sugar that results, not from eating sugar, but from insufficient levels of the hormone insulin, which maintains blood sugar (glucose) at normal levels. None of the various types of diabetes, including the more common type 2, type 1, and gestational diabetes, share the same cause, yet none is *caused* by eating sweet or starchy foods. Type 2 diabetes is caused by defects in either insulin secretion or its action, or in both. In other words, either your pancreas does not produce enough insulin or your body does not properly respond to the insulin it makes. This latter condition is referred to as insulin resistance. Insulin resistance is your own body's inability to use insulin efficiently, and it prevents your cells from getting enough sugar from your blood stream.

"When I was growing up food was my best friend, and I got into the habit of eating cupcakes, cookies, ice cream, and chips," Preston, a twenty-six-year-old health worker from Knoxville, told me. "My parents worked late and I was alone a lot; I grazed on sugar to take away the loneliness." When, at 300 pounds, Preston felt "crummy" enough to heed his sister's advice and go to the doctor, he discovered his blood sugar was 450 and he had diabetes. "I just wept and cursed all the sweet things I'd put in my mouth for so many years." Upon going to a dietitian, Preston learned that diabetes isn't caused by eating sugar, but because he ate so many sweets, they may have contributed to his insulin resistance, a precursor of type 2 diabetes.

In type 1 diabetes the immune system, which normally protects you from viruses and bacteria, attacks and kills the beta (insulin-producing) cells in your pancreas. Within months or a year, the body will produce either just a trace of insulin or none at all. The reasons why this happens are still unclear, but scientists think the causes may be genetic, with one or more environmental triggers. These may include stress, toxins, or a virus. Type 1 diabetes usually occurs in childhood, although you can get it at any age. And, yes, it is very common for patients with type 1 diabetes to mistakenly think they caused their diabetes by eating a sugary diet. A diabetes educator told me of a newly diagnosed man in her class who told her that he was certain he got diabetes because he'd eaten so many grapes the past few months.

The third most common form of diabetes is gestational diabetes. This form of diabetes is similar to type 2 diabetes, but it occurs only in women during pregnancy. According to the American Diabetes Association, gestational diabetes affects about 4 percent of all pregnant women, or about 135,000 women in the United States each year. The cause is unknown, but it's believed that hormones from the mother's placenta block the action of the mother's insulin. This causes the mother's blood sugar to rise.

How type 2 diabetes develops

When one eats sugar or starch, the blood sugar level rises and the pancreas releases the proper amount of insulin to keep blood sugar within the normal range. In someone with type 2 diabetes, the production and/or action of insulin is inefficient, so after eating your blood sugar goes up but doesn't return to normal levels. Clinicians look at diabetes not as a sugar problem but as an "insulin inefficiency." There is, however, an important caveat here: Even though eating sugar does not cause diabetes, "if you have the gene for diabetes, eating an excess of sweets, over time, may accelerate the onset of diabetes by overstressing your beta cells causing them to become compromised," says Dr. Gerald Bernstein, director of the Diabetes Management Program at Beth Israel Hospital in New York City. Bernstein also says that consuming too many calories

> ### *Tip to Make You Tops*
>
> *Diagnostic criteria for pre-diabetes*—A fasting plasma glucose test (blood test performed in the morning before you eat) shows that your blood glucose (sugar) reading is between 100 mg/dl and 125 mg/dl (5.5 mmol/l and 6.9 mmol/l). Or during an oral glucose tolerance test (OGTT) [you drink a sweet liquid containing glucose, and blood samples are drawn before and one, two, and three hours afterward], your two-hour glucose level is between 140 mg/dl (7.8 mmol/l) and 199 mg/dl (11 mmol/l).
>
> *Diagnostic criteria for diabetes*—Your fasting blood sugar is 126 mg/dl (7 mmol/l) or higher, or an oral glucose tolerance test shows two hours into the test a blood glucose of 200 mg/dl (11 mmol/l) or higher, and/or two random blood sugar readings are 200 mg/dl (11 mmol/l) or higher. [As of early 2009 the hemoglobin A1c (a value that reflects your average blood glucose, 24/7, over a two-to three-month period) is being proposed as the preferred diagnostic test for diabetes.]

and too much fat contributes to insulin resistance, which hastens the expression of the gene(s) for diabetes. Dr. Bernstein advises that if you are at risk for type 2 diabetes and like to eat sweets, you should make sure you get enough physical activity to burn off excess calories and keep your weight in check. This will help neutralize stress to the beta cells. If you have type 2 diabetes, you've probably already lost some beta cell function, but maintaining a proper weight and getting regular physical activity can help halt further loss.

If you don't have the gene for diabetes, then no matter how much sugar or fat you consume, you will not get diabetes, except there's a caveat here too: your age, says Dr. Bernstein. When you are eighty years old, your beta cells may not work quite the way they did forty years ago and may be unable to withstand the stress of too many sweets or too much weight as they once did.

Increased insulin resistance leads to type 2 diabetes

The onset of type 2 diabetes generally occurs after years of increasing insulin resistance. This early stage of insulin resistance is commonly called pre-diabetes, so named because it typically precedes type 2 diabetes. Studies show that most people with pre-diabetes develop type 2 diabetes within ten years.

During the early stage of insulin resistance, beta cells are still strong enough to overcome the present insulin resistance, but as insulin resistance increases, the pancreas attempts to secrete greater amounts of insulin, and beta cells become more compromised. Finally, the pancreas can't produce enough insulin to meet the demand, and blood sugars rise to the level identified as diabetes. The three greatest influences that cause insulin resistance and, as a result, the expression of the diabetes genes are being overweight, being sedentary, and being more than forty-five years old.

MYTH #2

I have to be overweight to get diabetes.

TRUTH: *Actually* about 20 percent of people who get type 2 diabetes are not overweight, nor are most people who get type 1 diabetes.

Most people associate type 2 diabetes with being overweight, and frankly, how could we *not* make this assumption when we consistently hear that obesity is a major cause of type 2 diabetes? What we don't often hear is that only about one-third of obese people in the United States get diabetes, as reported by the National Institutes of Health, and, approximately 20 percent of people who get type 2 diabetes are of "normal" weight. Although being overweight certainly tips the scales in favor of your getting type 2 diabetes, weight has no bearing in one in five cases. People who get type 1 diabetes tend to be either of "normal" weight or underweight when diagnosed. Why? Because type 1 diabetes is an autoimmune condition, not a weight-induced insulin-inefficiency condition, and, because people with type 1 diabetes produce nearly no insulin to ferry sugar from the blood stream into the cells, they excrete excess sugar and, with it, calories.

The high percentage of type 2 diabetes among slim populations such as the Japanese clearly illustrates that you do not have to be overweight to develop type 2 diabetes. Diabetes specialists agree that excess weight is only one cause of type 2 diabetes and that the underlying causes are extremely complex and still relatively unknown.

Obesity usually causes insulin resistance, which, as explained in Myth #1, leads to elevated blood sugars and often diabetes. "However," says Dr. Irl Hirsch, endocrinologist and holder of the Diabetes Treatment and Teaching Chair at the University of Washington School of Medicine in Seattle, "there are many other causes of insulin resistance besides obesity. I see this proven every day by the thin, insulin-resistant Asians I treat. Also, we now know that type 2 diabetes has numerous genetic markers, not one or two as previously thought."

Dr. Gerald Bernstein says that getting type 2 diabetes largely depends on both the type of genes you have *and* the metabolic links among glucose, fat metabolism, and insulin action. This mystifying metabolic interplay, says Bernstein, is one of the reasons why there is no imminent cure for diabetes.

Yet, scrolling through numerous chat boards and diabetes specialist and patient blogs, I saw just how prevalent this myth is. Many people wrote how confounded they were to get type 2 diabetes and not be overweight or, as this woman did, of genes trumping weight:

"YES!!! You don't have to be overweight to get diabetes! I'm five feet tall and weighed 103 pounds when I was diagnosed with type 2 diabetes. It runs in my family and none of us are overweight!" Jeff O'Connell, a writer for *Men's Health* magazine, weighing 220 pounds at 6 feet 6 inches, with 12 percent body fat and a 32-inch waist, wrote about his own disbelief when he discovered he had pre-diabetes. But, then, Jeff's slender grandfather and father both had diabetes.

Another theory—thin people may be fat inside

It is often said, "Just because you're thin doesn't mean you're healthy," and now there seems to be proof. Dr. Jimmy Bell, a professor of molecular imaging at Imperial College in London, explains that being thin doesn't mean you're not fat on the inside. Some doctors believe our visceral (internal) fat, which surrounds vital organs such as the heart, liver, and pancreas, though invisible to the naked eye can be just as dangerous as the subcutaneous (external) fat that bulges underneath our skin.

Further, it's believed that controlling weight with diet alone is more likely to create fat around our internal organs, whereas being active keeps fat away from vital body organs. Since 1994, Bell and his team have performed nearly eight hundred MRIs to create "fat maps" showing where people store fat. According to the data, people who maintain their weight through diet rather than exercise are likely to have major deposits of internal fat, even if they are otherwise slim. Most obesity experts agree that among the general population, people of normal weight who are sedentary and unfit are at greater risk for earlier mortality than overweight and obese peo-

---

Tip to Make You Tops

Dr. Louis Teichholz, chief of cardiology at Hackensack University Medical Center in New Jersey, says that even people with a normal body mass index (BMI), a standard obesity measure, can have surprising levels of visceral fat. Indeed, 45 percent of the women and 60 percent of the men scanned by Dr. Bell and his colleagues had normal BMI scores and excessive levels of internal fat.

ple who are active and fit. Dieting may keep you slim, but healthful eating, aerobics, and resistance exercise keep you slim, strong, and more resistant to disease.

Detecting and guarding against type 2 diabetes

The same risk factors for type 2 diabetes apply whether you are slim or heavy: a family history of diabetes, increased age, being in a high-risk ethnic group, poor diet, and lack of physical activity. A woman's risk increases if she's had gestational diabetes, has heart or blood vessel disease or has polycystic ovary syndrome. Unfortunately, many health care providers think "diabetes" only when they see a patient who fits the typical stereotype—obese and inactive—and therefore often neglect to check people of normal weight for pre-diabetes and diabetes. Dozens of people I've spoken with who had some of the classical symptoms of diabetes, yet were not overweight, were not initially tested for high blood sugar.

If you have any of the risk factors or any of the symptoms for type 2 diabetes, which include constant thirst, waking in the middle of the night to urinate, waking with a headache, fatigue, blood pressure of 140/90 or higher, a recurrent urinary tract infection, or neuropathy (burning or tingling sensations in your feet, hands, or limbs as a result of nerve damage), ask your doctor for a fasting plasma glucose (FPG) test and an oral glucose tolerance test (OGTT) to check for elevated blood sugar.

MYTH #3

I don't have to watch myself because my doctor says I have "just a touch of sugar" or I'm "only borderline."

TRUTH: *Actually*, if your doctor tells you that you have "just a touch of sugar" or "you're borderline," you probably have pre-diabetes. This puts you at greater risk for developing type 2 diabetes, so it should be closely monitored and managed.

Being told that you have "just a touch of sugar" or that you're "borderline" means your blood sugars are higher than normal but not high enough to be considered diabetes. Today the common term for this condition is pre-diabetes. Pre-diabetes is diagnosed by a fasting (before breakfast) blood glucose reading of between 100 mg/dl and 125 mg/dl (5.5 mmol/l and 6.9 mmol/l) or an oral glucose tolerance test where your glucose level two hours into the test is between 140 mg/dl (7.8 mmol/l) and 199 mg/dl (11 mmol/l).

Minor insulin resistance causes the elevated blood sugar levels of pre-diabetes and greatly increases the chances of developing diabetes. However, even though approximately 6–11 percent of people with pre-diabetes develop diabetes each year (and, if left untreated, most people with pre-diabetes go on to develop full-blown diabetes within ten years), you can lower your risk of getting type 2 diabetes by taking certain actions.

Tip to Make You Tops

According to an American College of Endocrinology (ACE) task force, about 60 percent of patients who have both impaired fasting glucose and impaired glucose tolerance develop diabetes within six years. Don't ignore high blood sugars.

Today approximately 57 million people in the United States have pre-diabetes. Although your physician may not pay it much attention, endocrinologists know that the same complications associated with type 2 diabetes, such as heart and blood vessel disease and kidney and eye disease, often occur during pre-diabetes. At the 2008 American Diabetes Association (ADA) Scientific Conference, Dr. Robert Sherwin of Yale University School of Medicine said, "Damage begins before glucose levels rise to a point where diabetes is diagnosed." Studies show that about 10 percent of people with pre-diabetes have diabetic eye damage and that people with pre-diabetes have one and a half times greater risk of heart disease and stroke. Most internists and endocrinologists agree that pre-diabetes is not taken seriously enough.

I've interviewed many people with type 2 diabetes who, looking back, realized their doctor had told them years before they got diabetes that their sugars were a little high but didn't impress upon them the value of making changes. Bill, at thirty-two years old and 290 pounds, had pre-diabetes. He was so busy working three jobs that he ate only one home-cooked meal a day and got all his other meals on the run. To get Bill to change his ways, his doctor finally had to say, "Bill, if you don't lose that weight you'll die a young man." Over the next seven years Bill lost eighty pounds. Unfortunately, he regained them, and only when suffering from unbearable fatigue did he go back to his doctor to hear him say, "Bill, you have diabetes."

The Diabetes Prevention Program

Pre-diabetes should be considered an alert: Make certain lifestyle changes now and you may avoid type 2 diabetes. The Diabetes Prevention Program, a landmark medical trial conducted in 1992 with over 3,000 participants, proved that moderate weight loss and exercise reduced by 58 percent the chances that someone with pre-diabetes would develop type 2 diabetes. In people aged sixty and older, the risk was reduced by 71 percent! People who lost 5–10 percent of their body weight, walked thirty minutes a day five days a week, and received intensive education and support proved that these measures were more effective at reducing the risks of developing type 2 diabetes than the measures taken by a control group that treated their diabetes by taking the glucose-lowering medicine metformin (brand name Glucophage®) and made few lifestyle changes.

If you still think that having "just a touch of sugar" is nothing to be concerned about, take a look at how the ADA's guidelines have changed over the years to characterize diabetes. Only a few years ago, the ADA's definition for diabetes was a fasting blood sugar of over 180 mg/dl (10 mmol/l). Then it was changed to above 140 mg/dl (7.7 mmol/l). Now it is 126 mg/dl (7 mmol/l) or higher. Some recent studies indicate that it should be lowered to 100 mg/dl (5.5 mmol/l). New guidelines from the ADA also say that many more people should get tested for pre-diabetes if they have any of the risk factors that follow.

Risk factors for pre-diabetes

- Over forty-five years of age
- Have diabetes in your family
- Regardless of age, if you're overweight and have a BMI over twenty-five
- Belong to a high-risk ethnic group, including Native Americans, African Americans, Latinos, Asian Americans, and Pacific Islanders
- Have a history of gestational diabetes or have delivered a baby that weighed more than nine pounds at birth
- Have metabolic syndrome, characterized by high cholesterol and triglycerides, high LDL (bad) cholesterol and low HDL (good) cholesterol, obesity, hypertension, and insulin resistance
- Have polycystic ovarian syndrome (a disorder in females marked by lack of menstrual periods, unusual hair growth, and excess weight)

If your blood glucose levels are in the normal range, get checked every three years for pre-diabetes, and if you have it, get tested for type 2 diabetes annually.

Tip to Make You Tops

New imaging technology can pick up telltale signs of metabolic stress in the retina, indicating that a patient may have either pre-diabetes or diabetes. Tests are now in clinical trials.

Detecting and managing pre-diabetes
before it becomes diabetes

First, find out whether you have pre-diabetes by having both a fasting plasma glucose test and an oral glucose tolerance test performed. If the results are not conclusive, it's recommended that you have one of these tests repeated on another day.

If you do have pre-diabetes, the first line of treatment is not medication but lifestyle changes. If you're overweight, losing approximately 5 percent to 10 percent of your body weight and engaging in moderate-intensity physical activity, such as walking or swimming two and a half hours each week, may return your blood sugar level to normal. Ask your health care provider to send you to a nutritionist or a diabetes clinic to learn more about healthful eating. You can also check out community resources such as the YMCA or a senior center for nutrition and exercise programs that may be offered free of charge.

If these measures are not sufficient to control your blood sugar or other complications of pre-diabetes, certain medications may then be advised. (For further information about medications, refer to Myth #15: Diabetes medications make you gain weight.) Finally, encourage family members to get screened; if you have pre-diabetes, they may too.

Type 2 diabetes is not as serious as type 1.

TRUTH: *Actually*, type 1 and type 2 diabetes are equally serious, because they both can lead to the same devastating complications.

Medical professionals will tell you that both types of diabetes are serious because they can cause the same debilitating and life-threatening diabetic complications, including heart attack, stroke, nerve damage, kidney failure, blindness, amputation, gastro-paresis, and sexual dysfunction. Although type 1 and type 2 diabetes differ in their causes, treatments, and typical ages of onset, both conditions share a lack of insulin efficiency. In both cases, elevated blood glucose levels over time can damage large and small blood vessels throughout the body, resulting in complications.

People with type 2 diabetes are equally prone to complications

Barry got type 2 diabetes in his thirties. After a short burst of enthusiasm that involved following a healthful diet and getting regular physical activity at his tree-trimming business, he fell back into his old unhealthful eating habits and traded in his electric saw for an electric typewriter at a desk job. Within five or six years Barry's doctor put him on one oral medication, a few years later he added a second, and, approaching fifty, Barry started taking insulin before

---

Tip to Make You Tops

LuAnn got type 1 diabetes when she was just twenty-two months old. Doctors told LuAnn's parents that she would be lucky to live to the age of eighteen. LuAnn is fifty-eight years old today. "From the time I was old enough to understand, doctors have preached to me that complications arise from poorly controlled diabetes and the importance of taking good care of myself," said LuAnn. She heeded their advice and has suffered few complications.

---

each meal. In his most recent decade of living with diabetes, Barry's blood sugars have been nearly picture-perfect, but earlier neglect caused Barry, over the past seven years, to have open-heart surgery and to develop neuropathy in both feet so painful that he can't walk much anymore. "I know this is from my sugars not being in control in the beginning," Barry said. "During that time, in fact, twice they found me out here in my yard in a semi-coma. I wasn't behaving then or checking my blood sugars like I do today."

Kristin, a petite, soft-spoken woman, came up to me after I spoke to her diabetes support group, asking, "If I start taking insulin, can I ever stop?" Even though, like Barry, Kristin had had quadruple bypass surgery as a consequence of not managing her diabetes, she still didn't understand the importance of managing her blood sugars. "In the beginning," she said, "my doctor gave me pills and told me about diet and exercise, but I never had the time."

Of the more than one hundred people with diabetes I've spoken with, those who had years of not managing their diabetes well, whether they have type 1 or type 2, generally had some complications, whereas those who managed it well generally suffered few or no complications. The exception was among people who got type

---

Tip to Make You Tops

The American Diabetes Association recommends blood sugar levels between 70 and 130 mg/dl (3.9 and 7.2 mmol/l) before meals, blood sugars less than 180 mg/dl (10 mmol/l) two hours after starting a meal, and an A1C—a blood value that reflects average blood sugar for the past two to three months—under 7 percent, or as close to normal as possible (4–6 percent) without incurring hypoglycemia (low blood sugar). The Association of Clinical Endocrinologists recommends tighter control: blood sugars under 110 mg/dl (6.1 mmol/l) before meals, blood sugars lower than 140 mg/dl (7.8 mmol/l) two hours after beginning a meal, and an A1C of 6.5 percent or less. Dr. Richard Bernstein, who advocates the maintenance of near normal blood sugars for people with diabetes, if at all possible, recommends a blood sugar of 83 mg/dl (4.6 mmol/l) most of the time and an A1C between 4.2 and 4.6 percent—the lower end of numbers found in people who don't have diabetes.

---

1 diabetes more than four decades ago, before blood-testing meters were available. Yet it seems that for each of these individuals, I've met someone who has lived with type 1 diabetes and, through the good fortune of her or his genes and discipline in managing diabetes, has lived a long life with relatively few complications.

The secret to living a longer, healthier life

Authors Sheri Colberg PhD, an exercise physiologist, and Dr. Steven Edelman write in their book *50 Secrets of the Longest Living People with Diabetes* that the lessons learned from long-living people with both type 1 and type 2 diabetes are similar and apply to everyone. The key secret is strict control of your blood sugars to help prevent diabetic complications.

Perhaps the best living examples that type 1 diabetes is not more serious than type 2 are the Cleveland brothers, who both got type 1 diabetes, Robert at the age of five and Gerald at the age of sixteen. Today they are eighty-eight and ninety-two, respectively, and both have had accomplished careers and full family lives. Each has some minor complications—among them mild neuropathy and trigger fingers—and both are still active. Inheriting a good set of family genes undoubtedly has something to do with the extended longevity of these brothers, but Drs. Colberg and Edelman write that what has helped these brothers just as controlling their disease is their vigilance, hard work, self-sacrifice, and determination.

The emotional toll of diabetes affects people with both type 1 and type 2

Another issue that doesn't discriminate between type 1 and type 2 diabetes is the emotional burden—the hardship of unending management tasks and the frustration, worry, anger, burnout, and depression that afflict many people with diabetes. Diabetes demands an enormous amount of attention, continual work, and resilience, even when your results don't seem commensurate with your efforts.

People with both type 1 and type 2 diabetes are also at higher risk for depression than the general population, two to three times higher, clinical psychologist Susan Guzman says. "People are especially susceptible to depression from how overwhelming diabetes may seem and how different it can make you feel. It's also easy to feel I'm not doing it good enough or experience increased frustration, shock, and sadness if you get a complication."

In the end, all you need to know is that diabetes is serious, whether you have type 1 or type 2, and that managing it responsibly is the best protection against it becoming *more* serious.

MYTH #5

I've just been diagnosed;
I can't have complications yet!

TRUTH: *Actually* you can. More than 25 percent of all newly diagnosed type 2 patients have complications, as do some patients with type 1 diabetes.

At the time of diagnosis, as many as 25 percent of patients with type 2 diabetes have diabetic complications, including nerve damage, retinal (eye) changes, heart disease, and early signs of kidney damage. The reason is simple: Many people live with either type 2 diabetes or pre-diabetes for years before they're diagnosed. During this time, elevated blood sugars are damaging large and small blood vessels.

Today, of the nearly 24 million people with diabetes in the United States (250 million worldwide), an estimated 6–7 million, or one-quarter to one-third (a figure derived from applying diabetes prevalence estimates to data collected from multiple national health surveys) are undiagnosed. In addition, many of the at least 57 million U.S. adults who have pre-diabetes don't know they have it. Many people learn that they have diabetes only after a complication brings them into their health care provider's office. Problems with feet or vision are common early complications of diabetes.

Most children and adolescents with type 1 diabetes don't have diabetic complications when diagnosed because type 1 diabetes usually comes on abruptly, within a matter of months. Because of its quick onset, type 1 diabetes doesn't have a pre-diabetes phase in this age group. Even though patients don't tend to have chronic complications, some do exhibit acute symptoms such as ketoacidosis, a condition of high blood sugar and dehydration, where acid builds up in the blood. However, type 1 diabetes in adults is often marked by a slower onset preceded by years of high blood sugars. Adults are more vulnerable to some complications associated with type 2 diabetes, such as retinopathy, which usually appears as blurred vision.

Seth, an optometrist, got type 1 diabetes at twenty-six and was diagnosed because he couldn't see the ball at the end of the pool table!

Seth was experiencing the typical symptoms of type 1 diabetes (constant thirst, frequent urination, and losing weight), but his busy third year of optometry school kept him from seeing his doctor.

"There was a break room on the seventh floor of the medical building, and I was playing pool one day and said to my buddy, 'I can't see that ball at the end of the table.' He said jokingly, 'What's with you, do you have diabetes or something?' It was like a light bulb went on. I had gone to four years of undergraduate school and had my bachelor's degree in biology. I had studied diabetes, but when it's happening to you, you don't put it together. I told a clinical professor my symptoms, and he told me to get some test tape and urinate on it. I did, and when he heard the results, he told me to get a blood test. Sure enough, it was diabetes."

Typical early complications of type 2 diabetes

Thirty-nine years ago Ted, now a very active senior, was driving home from a business trip when he realized he couldn't read the street signs; he thought he was going blind. The next day, when asked to read the eye charts in his ophthalmologist's office, he said, "What charts?" His ophthalmologist made an appointment for Ted to see his primary care physician, telling him you don't become nearsighted this quickly without a reason. A urine test proved him right: Ted had diabetes.

Kathy Spain, a certified diabetes educator and registered nurse, diagnosed her own father with type 2 diabetes when he told her his foot was numb and hurt. Noticing that his big toe was red, she tested his blood sugar and found it to be high. The appropriate blood tests that followed confirmed her diagnosis.

Spain also says that many people who come into a hospital with a heart attack go home on insulin and with a diagnosis of type 2 diabetes, having lived with undiagnosed diabetes or pre-diabetes for years. Heart disease is a leading complication of diabetes, says Spain, but even if you're in a hospital with a heart attack, diabetes can go unnoticed. Ask those treating you to look for it.

Tests for detecting complications upon diagnosis

If you're diagnosed with diabetes, or with pre-diabetes, your doctor should have you take some or all of the following tests to check for complications. (For target values on the following tests, refer to Myth #20: If my diabetes is under control, there's no need to see my doctor.)

- Blood pressure reading—If too high, can lead to heart disease or stroke and cause damage to kidneys and eyes
- Cholesterol and triglyceride test—If too high, can lead to cardiovascular disease
- Electrocardiogram—To check the health of your heart

- Microalbumin test—To check for microalbuminuria (protein in the urine), which can lead to kidney disease
- Dilated eye examination—To check for diabetic retinopathy
- Foot exam—Detects poor circulation to the feet and peripheral neuropathy (nerve damage)
- Ankle-brachial index—To detect peripheral vascular disease
- THS test—Blood test to detect hypo-and hyperthyroidism, autoimmune conditions associated with type 1 diabetes
- Anti-gliadin IgG, anti-gliadin IgA, anti-endomysial, or anti-tissue transglutamine assay—Blood tests to detect possible celiac disease, an autoimmune digestive disorder associated with type 1 diabetes

Keeping complications from progressing

If you have complications upon diagnosis, chances are they're in the early stages. To keep them from progressing and possibly to prevent additional complications, monitor these functions closely.

Blood sugar—Tight blood sugar control is the single best way to reduce your risk of complications. Getting an *HbA1c test* and keeping your A1C percent below 7 as recommended by the ADA, or below 6.5 as recommended by the American Association of Clinical Endocrinologists, reduces the risk of diabetic complications by 35–40 percent.

Blood pressure—According to the ADA, blood pressure of less than 130/80 mmHg reduces the risk of cardiovascular disease (heart disease or stroke) by 33–50 percent. High blood pressure can be controlled with several FDA-approved medications.

Cholesterol—Aim for LDL less than 100 mg/dl (if at risk for heart disease, less than 70 mg/dl), HDL greater than 45 mg/dl,

---

Tip to Make You Tops

In 2008 a mathematical formula was derived to help translate A1C values into the units that match the numbers you get when testing with your glucometer, whether that's milligrams per deciliter (mg/dl), as used in the United States, or millimoles per liter (mmol/l), as used outside the United States. This value is called the estimated average glucose (eAG), and the hope is that using it will help patients better see the difference between their individual meter readings and how they are doing with their glucose management overall. The ADA added the eAG to its January 2009 Standards of Care, and increasingly, as health care providers become familiar with it, the eAG will be given to patients alongside their A1C value.

---

and triglycerides (blood fats) lower than 150 mg/dl, can reduce cardiovascular complications by 20–50 percent. Statins are a widely prescribed medication if diet and exercise are not enough. If you suffer from muscle weakness due to statins, the supplement coenzyme Q10 (available at health food stores) may relieve symptoms.

Eyes—Treating diabetic eye disease with laser therapy can reduce the development of severe vision loss by an estimated 50–60 percent. Laser surgery does not reverse the damage in most cases of diabetic retinopathy, but it can prevent further vision loss.

Feet—Comprehensive foot care programs can reduce amputation rates by 45–85 percent. There are also medications to alleviate the pain of peripheral neuropathy in the feet and to improve circulation to the area.

Kathy Spain, Certified Diabetes Educator

Five Ways to Take Care of Your Diabetes

1. Test, test, and test your blood sugars again—if you don't test it is difficult to determine how best to manage your diabetes. Test your blood sugar at different times of the day, including two hours after the start of a meal. It is not enough to test only first thing in the morning.

2. Exercise even if you cannot do the recommended thirty minutes, five days a week—a little is better than nothing and can improve your numbers.

3. Never skip your medication unless it's approved by your doctor. If you experience side effects, talk to your doctor. There are many different medications that can be tried. If finances are a problem, ask your health care provider for information on assistance programs.

4. Be diligent about carbohydrate-counting: Occasionally measure your portions out so you can see what the correct portion size is. If blood sugars are normal, don't get lazy and think this means you are cured of your diabetes. You still need to follow your diabetes management plan.

5. See your doctor every three months to go over your blood sugars, to be examined for potential complications, and to make changes as needed to your diabetes management plan. Have your lab work done a week before your scheduled visit, so you can go over the results with your physician. Schedule your next visit before you leave the office.

Kidneys—Detecting and treating kidney disease early can reduce decline in kidney function by 30–70 percent. Maintaining tight control of blood glucose reduces the risk of kidney disease by 21 percent, according to results of a study reported at the 2008 annual meeting of the American Diabetes Association. In patients with early stages of kidney damage, renal function may be preserved using a class of drugs called ARBs and ACE inhibitors. The members of a newer class of drugs called renin inhibitors show similar kidney protection.

MYTH #6

Only adults get type 2 diabetes and only kids get type 1.

TRUTH: *Actually*, type 2 diabetes is occurring in children at an alarming rate, and you can get type 1 at any age.

The rise of obesity in children now makes them the newest at-risk population for type 2 diabetes. Before 1994, only about 5 percent of school-age children were diagnosed with type 2, but today that rate has skyrocketed to between 30 and 40 percent, and the use of insulin in children rose 150 percent from 2001 to 2007. Type 1 diabetes, caused by the destruction of beta (insulin-producing) cells within the pancreas, occurs principally in children and adolescents but can, and does, occur at all ages. In fact, many adults who get type 1 diabetes are misdiagnosed with type 2 because type 1 is so strongly identified with youth. Little more than a decade ago, type 1 diabetes was called "juvenile diabetes" and type 2 "adult-onset diabetes." The names were officially changed in 1997 to type 1 and type 2 diabetes to more aptly reflect the fact that age is no longer as dominant a factor.

The rise of type 2 diabetes in children

What is causing the rise of type 2 diabetes in children? In a word, obesity. About 95 percent of children with type 2 diabetes are overweight or obese when diagnosed, and obesity has shrunk the cycle time for developing both insulin resistance and type 2 diabetes. It used to take decades to develop insulin resistance as adults put on extra pounds; that's precisely why type 2 was commonly diagnosed in adults over the age of fifty. However, with so many children now severely overweight, that cycle time has been dramatically shortened.

With the rate of obesity now three times higher than in the 1970s, it is likely that one in every three American children born in 2000 or thereafter will be diagnosed with diabetes in their lifetime, and it is anticipated that in the next fifteen years, the global incidence of type 2 diabetes in children will increase by up to 50 percent.

Warning signs of type 2 diabetes in children

The symptoms of type 2 diabetes in children aren't always obvious. Diabetes often develops gradually, and about half of all children with type 2 diabetes do not have any symptoms at all. A diagnosis is often made when a child is screened for other disorders related to obesity. However, if there are symptoms, they are usually mild and may include

- Increased thirst and frequent urination
- Extreme hunger
- Weight loss
- Fatigue
- Blurred vision
- Acanthosis nigricans—Light-brown-to-black markings usually on the neck, under the arms, or in the groin

Risk factors for developing type 2 diabetes

If you think your child has the symptoms of diabetes or a risk factor listed below, ask your doctor to do a simple blood test to check.

- Overweight and sedentary
- High-risk ethnic group—African Americans, Latinos, Native Americans, and Asian Americans
- Family history—it's estimated that 45–80 percent of children with type 2 diabetes have at least one parent with diabetes
- High cholesterol and triglycerides
- High blood pressure
- The mother had gestational diabetes while carrying the child
- The child was either particularly large or particularly small at birth
- Polycystic ovarian syndrome

Type 1 diabetes in adults

Type 1 diabetes occurs in one out of ten people with diabetes, and although type 1 occurs most frequently in children, it also occurs in adults. Eugene J. Barrett, MD, former president of the American Diabetes Association and professor of internal medicine and pediatrics at the University of Virginia Health System in Charlottesville, says that in older people symptoms typically develop over four to five years, whereas in children diabetes seems to happen almost overnight.

Type 1 diabetes often comes on more slowly in adults, because they tend to have residual insulin production for several years. (I was told that, having developed type 1 at eighteen, I'd probably

---

Tip to Make You Tops

The symptoms of type 1 diabetes are the same in adults as in children: high blood sugar, excessive urination, hunger, thirst, and fatigue. Although adults with type 1 are often misdiagnosed with type 2 because of their age, they are not typically over-weight and do not usually have insulin resistance—the hallmark characteristics of type 2 diabetes.

---

begun to lose beta cell function around age twelve.) Genetics is a prime risk factor, but in many cases it's not a dominant one; many people with type 1 diabetes are the only one in their family with it. Environmental triggers are thought to be a primary cause of type 1 diabetes in adults, just as in children. If you're wondering how old you can be and still be diagnosed with what was once called "juvenile diabetes," the answer is that people as old as eighty have been so diagnosed!

My friend Phyllis got type 1 diabetes at age fifty-eight, and a lot of confused emotions came with her diagnosis. "I felt I'd been punched in the stomach," said Phyllis. "I had taken care of myself my whole life, I ate healthy, and I went to the gym. When I got diagnosed I kept asking, 'Why? What did I do?' But they don't know why I got type 1 or why I got it at that age."

With no real symptoms except extreme fatigue one weekend, Phyllis saw her doctor, and a blood test showed her blood sugar was 790! Because of her age, the doctor assumed she had type 2 diabetes and put her on pills, which didn't bring down her blood sugar. A week later she went to an endocrinologist, who diagnosed her with type 1 and started her on insulin. Two years later, Phyllis three times had to show her insurance company proof that she had type

1 diabetes in order to get them to cover her insulin pump. They didn't believe someone that old could have just gotten type 1!

Another type of type 1: LADA

Another form of type 1 diabetes that typically occurs after the age of twenty-five or thirty is latent autoimmune diabetes in adults (LADA). LADA is a slow-onset form of type 1. Patients are able to manage relatively normal blood sugars for several years with meal planning and oral medication because their loss of insulin production is slow, yet they will eventually produce little or no insulin. It is thought that as many as 20 percent of patients diagnosed with type 2 diabetes actually have LADA.

Yet another type of diabetes, which is known as "type 1.5," "double diabetes," or "hybrid diabetes," has characteristics of both type 1 and type 2 diabetes and can occur at any age. This happens when a type 1 patient becomes overweight and then develops the characteristics of type 2 diabetes, including insulin resistance, high blood pressure, and abnormal cholesterol and triglycerides. It also occurs when a type 2 patient develops antibodies to the islet cells of the pancreas and stops producing insulin.

Sadly, this form of diabetes can also occur in children, as was discovered in a five-year study performed by the National Center for Chronic Disease Prevention and Health called the SEARCH for Diabetes in Youth Study. Results showed that 30 percent of the children with type 2 diabetes had an autoimmune component to their diabetes (a characteristic of type 1 diabetes) and 30 percent of the children with type 1 diabetes were overweight (a characteristic of type 2).

If I have to go on insulin, it's the beginning of the end.

TRUTH: *Actually*, it's the beginning of achieving better blood sugar control.

The renowned Joslin Diabetes Clinic in Boston puts their type 2 patients on insulin immediately upon diagnosis. Angela Youngers, a diabetes educator and nurse practitioner who works at a Joslin satellite center, told me, "It's our first treatment because it provides the greatest control of blood sugars." Many people associate going on insulin with worsening diabetes, or they believe insulin causes complications. Neither is true. Diabetes tends to be, for most people who don't take care of it, and unfortunately for some who do, a progressive condition—over time your body produces less insulin, and/or your ability to use the insulin you do produce decreases. Far from being "the beginning of the end," for most people starting insulin is the beginning of better health.

Initial treatment of type 2 diabetes is typically diet and exercise and sometimes an oral medication to help control blood sugar. Usually within a few months or a few years, more medication is needed to keep blood sugars in the normal range, and one or more pills are added. As beta cells further degrade, more pills are added and then, for many patients, insulin. This successive course of treatment is designed to manage increasing insulin resistance as your pancreas becomes less able to meet the demand for insulin.

Increased insulin resistance is typically caused by obesity and a sedentary lifestyle; however, genetics, certain medications, and some other diseases (such as polycystic ovarian syndrome) are also causal factors. More than 40 percent of patients with type 2 diabetes use insulin. Today, the scientific and medical communities, including the American Diabetes Association, recommend earlier intervention with insulin.

Many people also mistakenly believe insulin causes diabetic complications such as blindness, kidney failure, and amputation, possibly because they've seen a loved one suffer such consequences shortly after beginning insulin therapy. But these patients' complications result not from using insulin, but rather from prior years of uncontrolled blood sugars.

Tip to Make You Tops

Many patients are prescribed premixed insulin, which is a combination of both rapid-acting and longer-acting insulin. Although premixed insulin is more convenient to use, it's not as effective for meeting glucose targets and losing weight. A diabetes educator can help you design a treatment plan that includes the proper insulin(s) for meeting your needs. To locate a diabetes educator in your area, call the American Association of Diabetes Educators at 800-338-3633, or visit their Web site: www.diabeteseducators.org.

Insulin's benefits and side effects

The benefits of using insulin are both short- and long-term. Short-term advantages include better blood sugar control which

---

Tip to Make You Tops

I know countless patients who feel so much better after adding insulin to their treatment plan that they wish they had done so sooner. Frank, who'd always been an avid horseback rider, was finally able to return to riding, once insulin helped stabilize his blood sugars. Gerry's years of up and down blood sugars—which caused fatigue, irritability, irrational decision making, and anger—cost him his business and almost his family, until he began using a long-acting insulin. Charles, who got diabetes at seventy, says, "I was sure insulin would keep me from doing the things I love like fishing, so I told my doctor I wouldn't do it. But he pressed and so I started it. I had better blood sugar control within weeks and haven't missed a day of fishing." When her pills weren't giving her the control she needed, Joanne felt that she'd done something wrong and insulin was her punishment. But now that she is taking insulin, her A1C test results are always under 7 percent.

---

leads to feeling less fatigued, having more energy, clearer vision, sleeping through the night, and possibly halting or reversing complications. The long-term benefit of using insulin is a reduced risk of diabetic complications, including not only the ones already mentioned, but also heart disease, eye disease, neuropathy, circulatory problems, gastroparesis (slow stomach emptying), hearing loss, trigger fingers, and diabetic cheirarthropathy, a stiffening of the hands and fingers.

Although insulin doesn't cause the types of side effects that many oral medications do (such as nausea, diarrhea, upset stom-

LOOKING THROUGH THE LENS OF ...
Betty Brackenridge, Director of Professional Training, Diabetes Management & Training Centers, Phoenix

Five Ways to Take Care of Your Diabetes

1. Get clear about your reasons for controlling diabetes. Doing things just because your doctor says so won't last. Pursuing your own goals will.
2. Forget about guilt; diabetes is a disease, not a character flaw. You deserve a long, healthy life and credit for all you do.
3. Use blood glucose results to become the world's expert on *your* diabetes. Only testing can show you how to eat your preferred foods and live your preferred life without giving up diabetes control.
4. Learn what's needed to protect your health (such as yearly eye checks and quarterly lab tests) and ask for them. If necessary, demand them. Regular checks are the only way to find problems before they become dangerous.
5. Successful diabetes treatment is a journey, not a destination. When your control changes for no apparent reason, see your team. It's probably time for a change in medicines.

ach, and skin rashes), some people may experience diabetic lipohypertrophies. These are small depressions or raised lumps that appear at the injection site as a consequence of the loss or buildup of fat just below the skin's surface. This is due to repeated injections at the same site or at a cluster of nearby sites. In rare cases, one can be allergic to the preservatives in a particular insulin, and insulin can cause hypoglycemia (low blood sugar).

Why providers hesitate to put patients on insulin

Much of the reason why patients have come to believe that when their physician recommends using insulin it's "the beginning of the end" is the way insulin is often introduced—as a last resort. Unlike the Joslin clinics that prescribe insulin upon initial diagnosis, most clinics and physicians wait years—until beta cells are almost completely nonfunctioning—before putting patients on it. Diabetes educator Betty Brackenridge says the primary reason why more patients aren't put on insulin sooner is physicians' own lack of expertise with insulin and training in its use. Most medical students receive no more than one to two days of education on diabetes. Endocrinologist Irl Hirsch says that when he brings medical students to his clinic and shows them a vial of insulin, it's the first time that most of them have ever seen it. If you think insulin may help you better control your blood sugar, ask your doctor about it even if he or she hasn't asked you.

MYTH #8

So many of my family members have diabetes, I'm certain to get it!

TRUTH: *Actually,* you may be predisposed to getting type 2 diabetes, but you can do a lot to possibly prevent it.

I've interviewed many people who have a strong family history of type 2 diabetes: their mom, dad, aunts, and cousins all have it, and they're certain they will get it. Genetics is undoubtedly a strong predictor for getting type 2 diabetes, but lifestyle habits such as diet and physical activity can have just as much (if not more) influence on whether you get type 2 diabetes. Here's what the experts say: Even if you have a family history of diabetes, losing 5–10 percent of your body weight; getting thirty minutes of physical activity three to five days a week; and maintaining the recommended levels for blood pressure, cholesterol, and triglycerides can often delay or even prevent the onset of type 2 diabetes. Even if you have pre-diabetes, taking these steps can help you avoid getting diabetes.

It's true that type 1 diabetes is not currently preventable. Although there are a genetic component and environmental triggers, lifestyle factors do not appear to influence getting the disease. Scientists are working hard to better understand why the body attacks its own cells and are seeking ways to preserve beta cell function.

During gestational diabetes, which typically develops between the twenty-second and twenty-eighth weeks of pregnancy, you

---

Tip to Make You Tops

The Nurses' Health Study, the largest women's health study, with more than 120,000 women aged thirty to fifty-five, revealed that those who had a healthy weight (defined by a body mass index of less than twenty-five), ate a healthful diet, engaged in thirty minutes of daily exercise, did not smoke, and had about three alcoholic drinks per week were less likely to develop diabetes than those women who did not exhibit these lifestyle habits. A follow-up study found similar results for men.

---

become resistant to the effects of your own insulin. The best way to prevent gestational diabetes is the same as the best way to prevent type 2 diabetes: Maintain a healthful weight, get regular exercise, and keep your fat levels (cholesterol and triglycerides) and blood pressure in check. The good news is that gestational diabetes goes away after your baby is born. The bad news is that a great many women who get gestational diabetes develop type 2 diabetes within five years after giving birth and for many it's as a consequence of excess weight and lack of physical activity.

Genetics cannot be ignored—thin people get type 2 diabetes too. However, a lot fewer of them do, and health care professionals know that if you are overweight or obese and sedentary, you are far more likely (some say between twenty and forty times more likely) to develop diabetes than someone with a healthy weight who is active.

Know your risk factors for type 2 diabetes

In addition to excess weight and being sedentary, here are the common risk factors for type 2 diabetes:

- Having pre-diabetes (50 percent of people with pre-diabetes go on to develop type 2 diabetes)
- Being 45 or older
- Having family members with diabetes
- Having had gestational diabetes or a baby weighing over nine pounds at birth
- Having high blood pressure and high lipids (cholesterol and triglycerides)
- Smoking
- Drinking more than a moderate amount of alcohol
- Having sleep apnea–like symptoms

If you have one or more of these risk factors, see your doctor. Diabetes educators say your health care provider is likely to be able to offer you medicine, treatment, or guidance now that can help you prevent diabetes. You can also judge your risk by taking the Diabetes Risk Test on the American Diabetes Association's Web site, www.diabetes.org. I'm told that the only way to fail this test is to discover you're at risk for diabetes and do nothing about it.

Steps to take that can increase your chances of preventing type 2 diabetes

Today's society is a veritable Petri dish for developing type 2 diabetes—much of our food is overly processed, we consume too much of it, and we get little to no exercise. Here's a case in point to illustrate how our unhealthful habits have contributed to diabetes: Just fifty years ago, Native Americans had no tribal cures for diabetes because almost nobody had it. Today it's rampant on the reservation. Having moved away from their traditional diet of lean meat and fish, whole grains, and a small amount of fried foods, the calories from which they burned up working the land, Native Americans now have the highest incidence of type 2 diabetes of all ethnic groups. They clearly have a genetic predisposition, but it lay largely dormant until their new, unhealthful lifestyle habits created a diabetes tsunami.

Preventing diabetes means making more healthful choices, and you can start with the ones below. Diabetes educators and psychologists say the best way to adopt better habits is to work on one or two small things at a time that you think you can improve.

- Eat breakfast. Eating breakfast gets your metabolism going, which helps you burn more calories throughout the day. Skipping breakfast makes you hungry all day and more prone to night binging.
- Buy fresh food, cook at home, and freeze meals for the week.
- Firmly push food away when you're 80 percent full, and gently push away loved ones who want to love you with too much food.
- Use smaller plates—you'll put less on them.
- Cut regular soda out of your diet.

That super-size Coke at McDonald's and other fast-food chains has approximately twenty-six teaspoons of high-fructose corn syrup (sugar) in it. Not only is consuming too much sugar unhealthful, but many dietitians and food researchers accuse high-fructose corn syrup (found in dozens of products, such as ketchup, cereal, juice, muffins, and even toothpaste) of altering the way our metabolism works, affecting insulin production, interfering with how fat is stored, and tricking our bodies into craving more calories.

- Limit visits to fast-food restaurants to a once-a-week or once-every-two-weeks treat.
- Develop an exercise program involving an activity you like, and increase your effort gradually.
- Climb the stairs whenever you can.
- Park farther away from where you're going, or get off the bus one or two stops early, and walk the rest of the way.
- Take up yoga, stretching, or simple walking to relax and quiet your mind.
- Wind down before bed with a good book or some deep breathing, not the 11 o'clock news.

MYTH #9

People with diabetes can't eat sugar.

TRUTH: *Actually,* people with diabetes can eat anything, including sugar.

The days when sugar was off limits if you had diabetes are over. People with diabetes can eat anything, with the recommendation that you, like everyone else, are best served by adhering to a healthful diet. Today, the American Diabetes Association's recommended dietary guidelines are the same as those of the U.S. Department of Agriculture: Eat a well-balanced, nutritious diet that contains foods from all the major food groups; is low in fat, cholesterol, and simple sugars; and provides most of your calories from whole grains, vegetables, fruits, lean meats, healthful fats, and fiber. Hallelujah, there are no forbidden foods!

This notion that people with diabetes shouldn't eat sugar is one of the hardest myths to lay to rest, says Dr. John Bantle, professor of medicine at the University of Minnesota, in a June 2008 *Diabetes Health* article titled "Sugar and Diabetes: The Myth That Won't Die." Fifteen years ago, Bantle and his colleagues performed an experiment comparing two meal plans. Both had the same amount of carbohydrates, the food most responsible for raising blood sugar. In one meal plan the carbohydrates came primarily from sugar, and in the other primarily from starch. Participants ate the foods from one meal plan for twenty-eight days and then switched to the other meal plan. The researchers discovered that participants' blood sugar levels were essentially the same whether they ate the sugary meals or the starchy ones. Conclusion: Sugar and starch raise blood glucose equally. Thus it's the amount of carbohydrate, not the source, that determines blood glucose levels.

"Intuitively it makes sense that you shouldn't eat sugar," says Bantle, but starch is also a string of glucose molecules. The sweet desserts that end your meal (such as cake and pie) and the starchy foods that form your meal (such as potatoes and rice) are all carbohydrates and all raise blood sugar. "If you add dessert to a meal, increasing the amount of carbohydrate," says Bantle, "your blood sugar will be higher, but you'd have the same effect if you had a double helping of mashed potatoes or an extra roll."

Tip to Make You Tops

When my diabetes was diagnosed thirty-seven years ago and I was given a "diabetic diet," candy bars were definitely not on it. Today, however, I allowably indulge my sweet tooth several nights a week by savoring one or two small squares of really good dark chocolate. Not only is it delicious, but dark chocolate provides heart-healthy antioxidants.

How to work sweets into your meal plan

In its 2008 position statement, the ADA stated that sucrose-containing foods can be substituted for other carbohydrates in a meal plan or, if added to the meal plan, can be covered with insulin or other glucose-lowering medications. That means people with diabetes can eat desserts, use sweeteners, and still keep their blood glucose in their target range.

Here's a simple example of how to substitute two foods of equal carbohydrates. Most people's meal plan calls for about forty-five to sixty grams of carbohydrates at each meal. Let's say you'd like to have two cookies, which are equal to thirty grams of carbohydrate, the same as two carbohydrate exchanges. Your lunch is a turkey sandwich with two slices of bread. Because two slices of bread also equal about thirty grams of carbohydrate, you can make an exchange: Either skip the bread entirely and have the two cookies, or eat one slice of bread and one cookie. Your total amount of carbohydrates remains the same. This strategy of exchanging carbohydrates can be used at any meal. If you need help adjusting your medicine to accommodate adding carbohydrates, check with your health care provider.

How to moderate your carbohydrate intake

Even though we've been liberated from absolute "don'ts" when it comes to sugary foods, it's best to keep sweets to an occasional treat. The more you replace nutritious foods with sweets, the less healthful your overall diet will be, and you are bound to consume more calories and put on weight. Try these ideas to keep your sugar intake to a moderate level:

- Replace sugar in hot and cold drinks with a low-calorie sweetener.
- Choose sugar-free products that have a low carbohydrate content.

- Choose lower-calorie, lower-sugar versions of your favorite dairy products and desserts.
- Eat a small serving of your favorite dessert, instead of a bigger serving of something less satisfying.
- When you eat out, split desserts with others at the table.
- Skip ready-made hot chocolate and make Riva's Hot Chocolate instead: a teaspoon of unsweetened cocoa powder, ¾ mug of hot water, 1 tablespoon of half-and-half, and one Sweet'N Low packet.

The glycemic index ranks foods according to their effect on glucose levels

A way to *not* limit your carbohydrates and to choose healthier carbs is to eat more low-glycemic-index (GI) foods and less high-glycemic-index foods. High-GI foods turn into glucose quickly and include typical sweets and desserts, such as cake, candy, cookies, soda, fruit juice, and syrups. Faster-acting sugars are also found in refined food products—foods where the outer fiber of the grain has been removed—such as white rice, white bread, bagels, pita, pasta, many breakfast cereals, muffins, and bakery goods. None of these foods are excluded from what you may eat, but they usually contain fewer nutrients and will spike and subsequently drop your blood sugar rapidly.

Foods with a lower GI, such as whole grains, beans, lentils, fruit, yogurt, skim milk, vegetable juices, sweet potatoes, oatmeal, and nonstarchy vegetables like broccoli, asparagus, cabbage, cauliflower, spinach, and sprouts convert into glucose slowly, creating a smaller fluctuation in blood sugar that helps you feel fuller longer. Foods rated with a low GI are also recommended for reducing the risk of heart disease and may help with weight loss. One way to eat more low-GI foods and less high-GI foods is to replace:

- White and gold potatoes with sweet potatoes
- White rice with brown or wild rice
- White bread with 100 percent whole grain bread
- Packaged breakfast cereals with slow-cooking, steel-cut oatmeal
- Pasta and cous cous with any whole grain, such as bulgur, barley, millet, oats, or buckwheat

---

Tip to Make You Tops

Cooking pasta al dente, that is, to the point where it's no longer hard but is still chewy and firm, enables you to digest it slowly, which creates a slower rise in glucose. "You're pretty much turning a high glycemic food into a low glycemic food," says dietitian Maudene Nelson. Dreamfields, a new brand of pasta, has a 65 percent lower glycemic index than regular pasta and twice as much fiber, dramatically reducing its carbohydrate count. Try it—I have and it works!

- Starchy vegetables such as corn, turnips, and beets with non-starchy vegetables
- Sweets such as cake and candy with fresh and dried fruit
- Chocolate chip cookies with oatmeal raisin cookies

MYTH #10

Diabetes is the leading cause of blindness, heart attack, kidney disease, and amputation.

TRUTH: *Actually*, it's "poorly controlled" diabetes that can cause these outcomes.

It's no wonder even some of the most educated people with diabetes think complications are inevitable; every time you hear about complications, there's no distinction made between those who have well-controlled diabetes and those whose diabetes is poorly controlled. Those of us who manage our diabetes well are likely to enjoy a long and healthy life, says psychologist Dr. William Polonsky.

Even as I am writing this, an article in the *New York Times* has made its way through the diabetes community and landed on my desktop, twice. The article, which is titled "Diabetes: Underrated, Insidious and Deadly," says, "Diabetes . . . wreaks havoc on the entire body, affecting everything from hearing and vision to sexual function, mental health and sleep. It is the leading cause of blindness, amputations and kidney failure, and it can triple the risk for heart attack and stroke." John Buse, the American Diabetes Association President for Medicine and Science and Professor at the University of North Carolina School of Medicine, says that diabetes is "a disease that does have the ability to eat you alive. It can be just awful—it's almost unimaginable how bad it can be." Buse also says, however, that patients who are focused on their disease and who have access to regular medical care have a good chance of living out a normal lifespan without developing a diabetes-related disability. Confused? No, you just have to insert "poorly controlled" before "diabetes" whenever you hear or read the health ramifications inaccurately attributed to *anyone* with diabetes.

Tip to Make You Tops

The landmark 1993 Diabetes Control and Complications Trial (DCCT)—the major clinical study conducted from 1983 to 1993 on 1,441 volunteers with type 1 diabetes—proved that keeping blood glucose levels as close as possible to normal (the nondiabetic A1C value is between 4 percent and 6 percent) can slow the onset and progression of, and significantly reduce the risk of, eye, kidney, and nerve damage. In fact, the trial demonstrated that any sustained lowering of blood glucose helps, even if a patient has had a history of poor control—and the same holds true for type 2 diabetes.

The benefit of well-controlled diabetes is reflected in the numbers

The Diabetes Control and Complications Trial (DCCT) and follow-up studies show that intensive blood glucose control reduces the risk of the following complications by the following percentages.

- Eye disease—76 percent reduction
- Kidney disease—50 percent reduction

- Nerve damage—60 percent reduction
- Cardiovascular disease—42 percent reduction
- Nonfatal heart attack and stroke—57 percent reduction

The twenty-year United Kingdom Prospective Diabetes Study (UKPDS)—the largest clinical study of diabetes ever conducted, with more than 5,000 patients—proved that lowering blood glucose reduces microvascular and macrovascular (small and large blood vessels) damage in people with type 2 diabetes just as in those with type 1. Controlling blood glucose was found to reduce the risk of the following complications by these percentages.

- Retinopathy (eye disease) and neuropathy (nerve damage)—25 percent reduction
- Vision loss greater than—33 percent reduction
- Kidney disease—33 percent reduction
- Strokes greater than—33 percent reduction
- Diabetes-related deaths—25 percent reduction

The major conclusion drawn from the UKPDS was that life-threatening complications of type 2 diabetes can be reduced by more intensive management using existing treatments. For instance, lowering blood pressure to less than 130/80 mmHg significantly reduces strokes, diabetes-related deaths, heart failure, microvascular complications, and vision loss and reduces the incidence of cardiovascular complications. At the 2008 ADA Scientific Conference, a panel of experts agreed that keeping blood glucose levels at or near the current recommended target range—between between 70 mg/dl (3.9 mmol/1) and 130 mg/dl (7.2 mmol/1) fasting and less than 180 mg/dl (10 mmol/1) two hours after a meal with less than

140 mg/dl (7.8 mmol/1) being "normal"—reduces damage to the small blood vessels that causes kidney disease and eye damage, and that keeping one's A1C under 7 percent reduces the risk of complications by approximately 40 percent.

Keeping diabetes, not just blood sugar, well controlled reduces the risk of complications by the following percentages.

- Controlled blood pressure can reduce the risk of cardiovascular disease by 33–50 percent, the risk of microvascular complications by 33 percent, and the decline in kidney function in early kidney disease by 30–70 percent
- Control of blood lipids, HDL and LDL cholesterol, and triglycerides can reduce cardiovascular complications by 20–50 percent
- Detecting and treating diabetic eye disease with laser therapy can reduce the development of severe vision loss by an estimated 50–60 percent
- Comprehensive foot care programs can reduce amputation rates by 45–85 percent

One controversial finding came in 2008 from the ACCORD study conducted in more than seventy clinical sites across the United States with type 2 diabetes patients at high risk for heart attack and stroke. Aggressive efforts were used to lower blood glucose below an A1C of 6 percent to see whether a decline in the rate of heart disease could be achieved. The study was actually halted eighteen months early because of a higher rate of deaths (a 0.03 percent increase) than expected. Dr. Jay Skyler, associate director for academic programs at the Diabetes Research Institute, who has carried out clinical research for more than three decades, said that a 10 percent reduction in heart disease *was* seen during the study and that if it had run longer, the study may have shown that the deaths were not a result of tight control, particularly since the patients were elderly with long-standing diabetes. Other large studies have contradicted the ACCORD trial's death rate, and the ADA's recommendation for patients to maintain an A1C of less than 7 percent has not changed or been refuted.

Diabetes educator Dr. William Polonsky likes to say that well-controlled diabetes is the leading cause of "nothing." Here my opinion differs, although I'm sure he'd agree with me. Well-controlled diabetes results, for many people, in the freedom to expect a long and healthy life.

Most people who have diabetes eventually lose their feet.

TRUTH: *Actually*, the chances of losing a foot are very small if you take care of your feet, and your diabetes.

Foot amputation, along with kidney disease and eye damage, has decreased significantly over the last several years. Lower-extremity amputations per 1,000 people with diabetes peaked in 1996 and declined by half in 2003. "By taking proper care of your feet, wearing appropriate footwear, and getting regular foot exams, you can stop foot trouble before it starts," says Birgitta Rice, diabetes educator and foot specialist. Experts agree that with simple, preventive foot care practices *and* good blood glucose control, you can greatly reduce your risk of foot problems and amputation.

Rice knows of what she speaks, having lived with type 1 diabetes for forty-nine years without foot complications. My own podiatrist, Dr. Joseph Stuto, has told me over the last several years, "You're doing everything you can to avoid a foot problem; you walk, you're lean, and you keep control of your blood sugar. Don't worry, just keep it up." Like Rice, I've had type 1 diabetes a long time—thirty-seven years—and I have no foot problems.

Tests and treatments for foot problems

Your podiatrist can perform certain tests to check the health of your feet. The last time I was in Dr. Stuto's office, he was conducting ankle-brachial index (ABI) testing on his patients. ABI tests check ankle pressure against arm pressure to see whether there's any narrowing or blockage of the arteries that supply blood to the legs and feet (a condition called peripheral arterial disease). It's a simple, painless test that indicates whether you're at risk for circulatory foot problems. Such preventive tests can often ward off an amputation.

Rice told me a remarkable story of a man who was scheduled to have his toes amputated as a consequence of a severe rash (ischemic petechia) and impending gangrene. A few days before the surgery, excruciating pain in his feet brought this man to his primary care physician. His doctor taught the man the relaxation and biofeedback technique called WarmFeet® to relieve the man's pain: By measuring the temperature of the skin surface of his feet and focusing his mind to send healing warmth there, the patient measurably improved blood flow and circulation to his feet. This not only relieved the man's pain but also improved the skin and tissues of his foot so dramatically that the amputation was canceled.

Tip to Make You Tops

You can learn more about WarmFeet® on the Web site www.warmfeetkit.com, or call 763-785-4013.

Hyperbaric oxygen therapy (HBOT) has also been used to heal gangrene and prevent amputation. HBOT requires soaking your feet in highly oxygenated water for an hour or an hour and a half once or twice a day, for several weeks. This transports extra oxygen to oxygen-starved tissue, often causing the gangrene to disappear. Many scientists and physicians believe HBOT can offer dramatic improvements in wound healing, diabetic neuropathy, ulcers, burns, and other conditions in which poor circulation plays a role.

If a foot problem has gone too far, sometimes an amputation is the only way to restore function and health to the area; at that point an amputation can be a life-saving procedure. I've interviewed several people who, not surprisingly, live functional and happy lives with prosthetics. One woman in particular, Kathleen, who's had diabetes for fifty-four years and has lost both her legs to amputation over the last few years, is one of the most positive people I've ever met.

During a vacation in the Bahamas, Kathleen got a cut between her toes, and by time she came home it was infected. She went into the hospital and stayed off her leg for almost nine months, but that was the beginning of continual foot problems. One day she stepped on a staple, which then lay embedded in her foot for several hours because she couldn't feel it. After she had gone to a wound clinic for months with no improvement, a vascular surgeon amputated her big toe. "The toe next to it began going black and the pain was awful," Kathleen said, "so I called the doctor and told him, 'Take my leg off!'" And so he did. Kathleen was fitted with a prosthetic below the knee. Six months later Kathleen's other foot got caught under her wheelchair, which damaged her toe. Soon gangrene set in. This time her other leg came off.

"I drive. I dance. There's life after amputation," said Kathleen, who lost her first leg five years ago on her sixtieth birthday. "This year I'll be traveling in England [for] two and a half months. Then I'm going down the Nile, and later in the year I'm going to Turkey and Greece. To me, losing my legs was a blessing. I've [had] no more of the awful pain I had for so long, and," she chuckled, "I don't have to buy expensive shoes or have pedicures. I don't need to shave my legs. A few months ago I went to a dinner theatre with friends and I was sitting at the table and my prosthetic was killing me so I took it off under the table. At the end of the play I put it back on and got up and I realized I'd caught the tablecloth in my prosthetic and it was skidding off the table coming toward me as I walked away." Now we both laughed.

What to do when your foot's out of your shoe

- Wash your feet every day with mild soap and warm water. If you've lost some feeling in your feet, test the water temperature with your hand first to be sure it isn't too hot.

Tip to Make You Tops

Although it is recommended that you wash your feet every day in lukewarm water and mild soap, it's not recommended that you soak your feet. Soaking of any length puts you at risk for infection. A cut or crack in your skin provides an easy entry for bacteria. Dry, flaky skin (caused by a soak) prompts you to scratch your feet, and scratching can create the breaks in your skin that let in bacteria. If your physician or podiatrist recommends you soak your foot or toe (as in the case of HBOT), follow her or his instructions. Otherwise, keep your tootsies out of the dishpan.

- Check the skin of your feet every day for any sign of irritation, injury, or redness—if you have lost sensation in your feet, you may not feel small sores, breaks, or changes in your skin. Make foot checks a habit: For instance, check your feet each day just before or after you brush your teeth in the morning. If you spot any change, cut, or discoloration, see your doctor right away. If it's hard for you to see your feet, have a loved one check your feet weekly.

- Apply an unscented moisturizer on your feet and calves to keep the skin soft and moist, but don't put lotion between your toes and don't put your socks or shoes on while your feet are still moist. This creates a breeding ground for fungus.

- Trim your toenails straight across, not down at the corners. If you find an ingrown toenail, see your doctor right away.

- If you have sores or wounds, wearing white socks is a simple way to see whether there's any oozing or bleeding.

- Don't play doctor by using antiseptic solutions, drugstore medications, heating pads, or sharp instruments on your feet; trying to mend a problem yourself can make it worse.

- Keep your feet warm for optimal blood flow. Wear warm socks and shoes in the winter, and try not to get your feet wet in the snow or rain. If you do, dry your feet immediately. If your feet are cold at night when body temperature tends to drop, wear a pair of loose socks to bed.

- Don't walk around barefoot, outside or inside. Wear shoes or slippers in the house to avoid stepping on something sharp.

- Smoking and sitting cross-legged decrease the blood supply to your feet. Avoid doing both.

**Birgitta Rice, Pharmacist and
Certified Health Education Specialist**

Five Ways to Take Care of Your Diabetes

1. Nightly, massage a diabetic foot cream into your feet to rehydrate dry skin, soften calluses, and provide soothing warmth, but don't put it between your toes.
2. Do some easy foot exercises to help strengthen your feet, increase circulation, and relieve pain. Point your toes for a few seconds and then, using your pointed toes, write your name in the air.
3. Take daily walks. It aids circulation to your feet.
4. Follow a diet and exercise plan. It is a good place to start to care for your diabetes—and your feet.
5. Keep up to date on new diabetes research findings.

Insulin shots are very painful.

TRUTH: *Actually,* today's insulin injections typically don't hurt, and most patients report that they hardly feel them at all.

Today's syringe needles are so short and thin that when I take out a syringe and show it to a diabetes group I'm addressing, they're surprised—they can barely see the needle. The old inch-and-a-half, thick steel needle from years ago has morphed into today's super-short (5/16 inch), and super-thin (gauge 31) needle. You barely see it or feel it. When a diabetes family therapist showed me the steel needle that he had to boil and inject three times a day into his nine-year-old body forty-five years ago, I almost wept. Thankfully, we've come a long way. Most people today say that shots are practically painless; a common reaction after a patient's first shot is "That's it?" I take between three and six shots a day, based on how I'm eating and exercising, and I don't think twice about it.

If you've never had an insulin injection, you're probably picturing the shot you get at the doctor's office, such as flu, tetanus, or Novocain shots. Not only are those needles much bigger and thicker, but they also go into a muscle or vein where you'll feel pain. Insulin, on the other hand, is injected into the fatty tissue right beneath the skin, a pretty pain-free zone. What's more, the needles are coated with silicone, which makes them glide into your skin with little or no discomfort.

Alternatives to syringes

The most popular alternative delivery device to syringes is the insulin pen, which resembles a large, thick pen and houses an insulin cartridge. Insulin pens have a needle that is just as thin as those in today's syringes and even shorter (sometimes as short as 3/16 inch, or 5 mm). My friend Ruth prefers the insulin pen to syringes. Because it doesn't *look* like a syringe, she disassociates it from any notion of pain. Also, pens can't break the way glass insulin vials can. "Then too," she says, "I like that the pen makes a clicking sound as I dial my dose so I know I'm getting my exact dose. That was always a problem when drawing up insulin from a vial, especially in bad light." I know that struggle full well, from the early days when I would draw up my dose under a blinking fluorescent bulb in a stall of the ladies room, too shy to do it in public. Today I'll "shoot up" almost anywhere, including right at the table in a restaurant, just being discreet enough to be polite. After all, part of my mission is to educate others about diabetes, and how can I do this if I squirrel away out of sight just to take my medicine?

Tip to Make You Tops

Novo Nordisk's NovoPen® Junior (Novolog) and Eli Lilly's HumaPen® LUXURA™ (Humalog) enable you to dose half units. If you have problems with dexterity or vision, Clickfine® pen needles, which fit all insulin pens, simply click onto your pen and require no twisting.

Now, in all honesty, there are instances where you may feel some pain from an injection. If you inject into a muscle by accident, for instance, or if you have scar tissue built up from years of injections under your top layer of skin, you may feel a twinge. If you hit a nerve, you'll certainly feel a sting, and if you're reusing your syringe, the needle will dull a little each time you inject. You may also feel pain if you tense up when giving yourself an injection, and sometimes injecting cold insulin stings.

There are some simple solutions to take the sting out of injections.

1. Always use a new syringe. This is also a sanitary precaution and the best way to avoid infection.
2. Rotate your injection site. Not injecting in the same spot twice in a row will cause less scar tissue to develop.
3. Let your insulin come to room temperature before injecting.

Some people prefer one of two other insulin delivery devices: the insulin pump or a relatively new device called the I-Port™. Many people with type 1 diabetes, as well as some with type 2, wear an insulin pump, which is about the size of a pager and is often worn on a belt buckle or in a pocket. It feeds an ongoing drip of insulin into the body through a small, thin tube that is inserted into the skin via a needle. The needle is quickly plunged into the top layer of skin with an insertion device. This is usually a pretty painless process, though just as with syringes, there can be some slight pain at times. Many people prefer wearing a pump to taking shots; they feel they get better blood glucose control, and they feel the prick of a needle only once every three days, when they change the needle and tubing.

A fairly ingenious device called I-Port™, from Patton Medical Devices (www.pattonmd.com), eliminates the need for your syringe needle to prick your skin at all. It's a small round disc, 1.5

inches (38 millimeters) wide, that sits on the top of your skin. It has an insertion needle that guides a very small, short, flexible plastic tube (cannula) under your skin. When you inject your insulin, you put your syringe needle into the little rubber center of the I-Port™ disc, so the syringe never pricks your skin. The insulin goes directly into the cannula and then into the tissue below. If you take four injections a day, you'll trade in twelve injections for just one insertion of the I-Port™ over a three-day period. This delivery system can be a boon for children and anyone who's needle phobic. I-Port™ plans in late 2009 to release an inserter to help patients more easily insert the device.

Tip to Make You Tops

There is one insulin device on the market that uses no needle. I've never actually met anyone who uses this, but every so often I read or hear about the insulin jet injector. It looks like a big pen and emits a fine spray of insulin through the top layer of your skin by a high-pressure air mechanism. Insulin jet injectors are costly and not pain-free, so if you're interested, you might want to try out different models before you buy one.

MYTH #13

There's nothing I can do to prevent my kids from getting diabetes.

TRUTH: *Actually,* there's a lot you can do to increase the odds of preventing type 2, and some research suggests it may be possible to prevent type 1.

Up until a decade ago, the incidence of diabetes in children consisted almost entirely of type 1, but there is now a rising tide of type 2 diabetes in children. The causes of type 1 are still uncertain, as are preventive measures. Some studies suggest that in Caucasian populations, cow's milk may influence your chances of getting diabetes; children who have been exclusively breast-fed seem less likely to develop type 1 diabetes. Dr. Lois Jovanovič, clinical professor of medicine in the Division of Endocrinology at the University of Southern California–Keck School of Medicine, points out that cow's milk contains casein, a protein that a baby has not yet developed enzymes to break down, and this causes babies to develop antibodies that increase the risk of their developing diabetes. Some doctors recommend breast-feeding children who have parents or siblings with diabetes or using soy-based formulas.

Since 1994 the National Institutes of Health has been conducting studies to determine how to preserve beta cells to prevent diabetes. Some of these studies attempt to alter our immune response, and others aspire to strengthen resistance. An early trial testing whether diabetes can be prevented in children who have a family history of type 1 by giving them insulin failed. However, another trial is now testing this hypothesis using oral insulin.

Tip to Make You Tops

If type 1 diabetes is in the family, you should have your children screened annually. TrialNet, an organization dedicated to the study, prevention, and early treatment of type 1 diabetes, provides such screening. Go to its Web site at www.diabetestrial net.org. Also, be attuned to type 1 diabetes symptoms: thirst, weight loss, excessive urination, and fatigue. Infants can get type 1 diabetes too, and one sign is diapers heavy with urine.

The rise of type 2 diabetes in children

The incidence of type 2 diabetes has doubled over the last decade, largely as a result of childhood obesity. About 32 percent of U.S. children are overweight or obese, and one out of ten is considered morbidly obese. The article "It's Not Just Genetics" reports that over the past few decades, the entire American environment has become much more obesity-supporting, with an increasing supply of fast-food outlets where meal sizes have ballooned. Physical activity has been largely eliminated from the daily lives of children, who now entertain themselves with an array of sedentary electronic pastimes that didn't exist a generation ago. "The environmental factors are much more compelling toward obesity than they were thirty years ago," says William Dietz, director of the division of nutrition and physical activity at the Centers for Disease Control and Prevention (CDC).

The handwriting was on the wall more than ten years ago when, in 1997, an international committee sponsored by the American Diabetes Association recommended that the term "adult-onset" diabetes be changed to "type 2" diabetes because, as pediatric endocrinologist Francine Kaufman says, obviously type 2 was no longer limited to adults. Dr. Kaufman, head of the Diabetes, Endocrinology and Metabolism Center at Children's Hospital Los Angeles, is a tireless public advocate for preventing type 2 diabetes in children. In her book *Diabesity: The Obesity-Diabetes Epidemic That Threatens America—And What We Must Do to Stop It*, she writes that the incidence of type 2 diabetes in children is our next epidemic.

Dr. Kaufman says that all parents should become familiar with these early signs of high blood sugar:

- Wetting the bed and waking up at night to urinate
- Excessive thirst
- Weight loss
- Increased hunger
- Fatigue
- Sores that don't heal

African American families should also be alert for these symptoms of insulin resistance that may affect their preadolescent daughters: a darkening of the skin around the neck, in the crease of the arm, and the folds of the groin (a condition called acanthosis nigricans); an absence of their menstrual period; hair loss; and skin tags or little moles.

What you can do to help prevent type 2 diabetes in your children

Even though genetics plays a strong role in diabetes, if you have diabetes it doesn't mean your child will necessarily get it. Excessive weight and being sedentary are the most influential triggers for diabetes. Type 2 diabetes is as preventable in children as it is in adults, through maintaining a healthful diet and weight and being physically active. Prepare healthful meals for your children. Kids, just like adults, need a diet rich in fresh vegetables, fruit, lean protein, and low-fat dairy, with a minimum of sugar and fat. And get your kids away from the computer and TV screen. In 2000 the average child watched 40,000 commercials, double the number in 1970.

Most health educators say parents must also be role models for their children; *you* need to adopt a healthful lifestyle to set the right example before asking your children to do so. If you have older children, talk with them about diabetes and the value of being fit and eating healthy when they're out of the house. Putting children on the right track now can both help prevent childhood diabetes and reduce the risk that they'll develop diabetes as adults.

Tip to Make You Tops

If your child is struggling with his or her weight, help your child to make healthier everyday choices like eating healthier foods and smaller portions—rather than berate or nag your child to lose weight.

Practical steps to reduce your child's chances of getting diabetes

- Serve a healthful breakfast and whenever possible eat dinner together as a family.
- Cut back on, and then virtually eliminate, sugar-sweetened drinks, including juice.
- Serve more vegetables, fruit, and whole grains and less junk food. For dinner, fill half your child's plate with different-colored vegetables.
- Offer food options so your child doesn't feel deprived, but set limits. For instance, let your child choose among a small bowl of berries, grapes, or an orange for dessert.
- Save sweets for a weekly treat.
- Don't eat in front of the television, and don't let your kids do it either.
- Limit your child's TV watching and use of the computer to two hours a day.
- Have the whole family spend more time engaged in physical activities. Take your kids to the park, play Frisbee together, let them run around—kids need at least sixty minutes of moderate to vigorous physical activity per day.

Get involved in making your community healthy to help prevent diabetes

Our societal infrastructure, from families to schools to government, is where we all need to be looking to decrease the incidence of diabetes in children, says Dr. Kaufman. California led the way in 2003 by banning sugary sodas from public schools, and, in response to parental demand, various states across the country have followed suit. In Arizona, the Pima tribe of Native Americans, which has some of the highest obesity levels in the world, is growing school gardens in the desert to supply cafeterias with fresh vegetables. Today at least seventeen states have set nutritional standards for school meals that are stricter than those demanded by the U.S. Department of Agriculture. It takes a village and it takes concerned parents.

Tip to Make You Tops

Help arrange for a diabetes educator or person with diabetes to speak in your child's school. I know many children with diabetes who've addressed their classmates. Two years ago I spoke to a classroom of seventh graders at the request of their concerned health teacher, who wanted them to understand that making better food choices may help them prevent diabetes. All but three of thirty mostly African American and Hispanic fourteen-year-olds in his class had diabetes in their family. I showed them the difference in size and calories between a hamburger of twenty years ago and today's quarter-pounder with cheese and explained how a corn muffin has tripled in size and calories. We talked about how long they'd have to ride their bikes to burn off a slice of pizza. I told them what diabetes is like to live with and that they don't have to get it if they cut down on their carbohydrates and calories, get active, and watch the sugar and fat in their diet. When they left, a few kids actually shook my hand and thanked me! Maybe some really learned that day that there are actions they can take to help prevent diabetes.

Nicholas Yphantides, MD, is a family physician whose passion is creating communities that support health. Having reached his

Five Ways to Take Care of Your Diabetes

1. As your child takes more responsibility for her diabetes management, do not drop out of the picture altogether. From time to time, look at her blood sugar readings and remind her to test her blood sugar if necessary. You may even need to remind your child to take her insulin or other medication. Children with parents who remain involved in their care have better control of blood sugar levels.

2. Make sure your child sees her diabetes doctor every three months and has lab work done as recommended. Know what your child's hemoglobin A1c is.

3. Encourage your child to live as normal a life as possible, including participating in any activity she wants. Diabetes should not be used as an excuse to avoid exercise, which has a positive effect on blood sugar control.

4. Listen to your child when she says "I don't feel well." Oftentimes she will know when her blood sugars are out of range, even before the meter shows it. If your child says "I'm low," believe her!

5. Relax! Don't beat yourself up if you calculated the insulin dose or carb count wrong. Learn from your mistakes, and stay up to date on diabetes care so you can make informed decisions.

own intolerable weight of 467 pounds when he was only thirty, Yphantides lost 270 pounds and now co-chairs the San Diego County Childhood Obesity Task Force. This Task Force helped county and city governments create walking and cycling paths in existing communities. They campaigned for schools to provide students with both physical education classes and additional opportunities for sixty minutes of daily activity. They motivated one local school district to write a new policy to replace a number of high-sugar, high-fat snack foods and beverages available in vending machines with more healthful choices. If you're interested in learning more about making community improvements in the battle against obesity and childhood diabetes, go online to www.ccwsd.org.

If you have diabetes and you want to look for the silver lining, use your diabetes as a wake-up call for the whole family to make healthier choices that may prevent your children and other family members from getting diabetes. And take Dr. Kaufman's words to heart, because they're true for both children and adults: "If we could prevent obesity, type 2 diabetes would become rare."

MYTH #14

People who have diabetes have to wear special shoes.

TRUTH: *Actually,* you can wear any shoe that fits properly and doesn't put undue stress on your feet.

Because people with diabetes have to be especially careful in order to prevent foot injuries, shoes need a little extra consideration. But that doesn't mean you have to wear only one type of shoe or, for that matter, clunky, big, or ugly shoes. If you are not experiencing any loss of sensation in your feet, just be sure to wear proper-fitting and well-constructed shoes and have your feet measured before you buy new shoes; our feet tend to change in both size and shape as we get older. Joy Pape, foot care nurse and certified diabetes educator, says lifestyle changes may include some fashion changes, but if you know how to choose proper-fitting shoes, there are many good-looking options to protect your tootsies.

Here's what to look for in a shoe

- 3/8–1/2 inch of space between the end of your longest toe and the shoe. That's room enough for your finger to fit in the back of your shoe. Also see that you can wiggle your toes in your shoe.

- Shoes should be comfortable when you put them on—don't expect them to break in and stretch to fit your foot.
- Try to find shoes that have leather upper material and cushioned, comfortable insoles and soles.
- Avoid pointy-toe styles because they'll squeeze your toes.
- Shoes should be firm in the back to cradle and support your heels, yet not skin tight over the ball of your foot.
- If you want to wear heels, know that for every inch of height, the ball of your foot will endure 25 percent more pressure.

If you can't resist heels, limit your time in them. Pape advises us gals to wear flats until we get where we're going, put our heels on when we're there, and put our flats back on as soon as we leave. Ill-fitting shoes can cause many foot ailments, which, if you've lost sensation in your feet, you may not feel—from bunions, hammertoes, calluses, and blisters to wounds and sores. The best protective shoes will have deep toe boxes that prevent cramping and rubbing, a soft lining, and an absence of seams at critical spots inside the shoe.

Tip to Make You Tops

Under the Medicare Therapeutic Shoe bill, patients who qualify are entitled to one pair of special shoes and three sets of custom-molded inserts per year at an 80 percent discount. Qualifications include having diabetes and having had a foot problem; so check the guidelines to see whether you're eligible for coverage. You may also need a note or prescription from your foot specialist and general practitioner.

If your podiatrist recommends special shoes because you have a foot problem, follow his or her advice. A recent study of patients with foot problems who were at high risk for amputation showed that those who wore protective footwear had, as a group, far fewer amputations.

Many people, without realizing it, actually wear shoes that are too small for their feet. This usually happens either when you are not aware that your shoe size has changed or when you can't feel your feet and thus don't know your shoes are too tight. See whether there's a shoe store in your area that employs a pedorthist, a professional trained in the design, fit, and function of shoes and orthotics (a foot pad or heel insert custom-made or bought at the pharmacy that helps improve the health and function of the foot or ankle). A pedorthist will measure your feet and help you find a shoe with the correct shape and structure for *you*. The right shoe can redistribute pressure across the soles of your feet and help you walk better. Pedorthists are not a substitute for podiatrists, but sometimes they can help you alleviate a minor foot problem. A friend recently told me that the last time she bought new shoes she

---

Tip to Make You Tops

Shoe Do's
- Buy new shoes late in the day, when your feet are larger.
- Wear new shoes for only two hours or less at a time.
- Inspect the inside of each shoe before putting it on to make sure that nothing inside can irritate your foot.

. . . and Don'ts
- Don't wear the same pair of shoes every day.
- Don't lace your shoes too tightly or too loosely.

Joy Pape, Foot Care Nurse and Certified Diabetes Educator

Five Ways to Take Care of Your Diabetes

1. Look at your feet every day. If you look regularly at the top and bottom of your feet and in between your toes, you'll be familiar with how they normally look. If there is a change, you'll notice it right away and can get help before an unnoticed problem progresses and causes real trouble.

2. Don't go barefoot. This rule applies when you are at home, as well as outside. Most accidents happen at home, and wearing socks without shoes gives you no protection if you step on something or if something drops on your foot. Also, socks alone can increase your chance to slip and fall.

3. When you travel, it's tempting to bring new shoes, but be sure to bring a pair of old "comfies" as well. Many times people bring new shoes on a trip, walk more than usual, and then have foot problems.

4. Call your doctor right away if you have a problem. Most people who get serious foot problems do so by not calling their health care provider when they first notice a problem. Foot problems don't have to be big problems if you get help at the first sign of trouble.

5. The best you can do for foot problems is to prevent them by remembering your ABCs:

A = A1C	less than 7 or 6.5 percent
B = Blood pressure	less than 130/80 mmHg
C = Cholesterol (lipids)	
Total cholesterol	less than 200 mg/dl
Triglycerides	less than 150 mg/dl
HDL	In men greater than 40 mg/dl, in women greater than 50 mg/dl
LDL	less than 100 mg/dl, and less than 70 mg/dl if you have, or are at risk for, heart disease

worked with a pedorthist, who, when he measured her feet, saw that she had a callous under her middle toe. He recommended that she use a thin inner half-sole with some arch support to redistribute the pressure on her sole and explained that the callous should diminish. "Amazingly," she told me, "he was right. It went away in about two months."

Medical Myths

Diabetes medications
make you gain weight.

TRUTH: *Actually,* some do, some don't, and a newer class of drugs actually helps you lose weight.

Many older diabetes medications do cause weight gain. Among them are widely prescribed sulfonylureas, more commonly known as Diabinese® (chlorpropamide), Amaryl® (glimepiride), Glucotrol® (glipizide), and DiaBeta®, Glynase®, and Micronase® (glyburides). Prandin® (repaglinide) and Starlix® (nateglinide) also cause weight gain. All these medications stimulate the beta cells in the pancreas to produce more insulin to control blood sugar levels. Hypoglycemia (low blood sugar) and weight gain are the two most frequently reported side effects of these drugs: Hypoglycemia causes you to consume extra carbohydrates to raise your glucose, and it stimulates appetite.

Thiazolidinediones, more commonly known as Actos® (pioglitazone) and Avandia® (rosiglitazone), promote weight gain by triggering an enzyme that causes fat cells to enlarge by storing more fatty acids. Thiazolidinediones can also cause fluid retention, which increases body weight. Studies show that the gain is usually not more than five or six pounds.

By contrast, Glucophage®, the brand name for metformin, has been shown in clinical studies not to cause weight gain; it may even help manage weight or cause a small weight loss, on average four to six pounds. Metformin helps curb hunger by preventing the liver from producing extra, unneeded blood glucose, and it doesn't cause hypoglycemia. Adding Glucophage® to your regimen and cutting back on another oral medication may help limit weight gain. Januvia®, a newer oral medication, is weight neutral, and most patients find it easy to tolerate. Insulin may also cause weight gain—but not for the reason you think—and a newer class of drugs cause weight loss.

Tip to Make You Tops

Sudden weight gain from fluid retention can be a side effect of an oral diabetes medication, but it can also be a symptom of a number of serious underlying medical problems, including heart disease, kidney disease, high blood pressure, or even irritable bowel syndrome or celiac disease. Discuss any sudden, unexplained, or significant weight loss or gain with your health care provider.

Medications that promote weight loss

Byetta®, the first in a new class of drugs called incretin mimetics (drugs that mimic the effect of certain gut hormones), improves the body's ability to manage glucose levels by stimulating insulin production; inhibiting the liver from secreting glucagon, a hormone involved in carbohydrate metabolism; and slowing stomach emptying, which makes you full faster. Byetta® has been proved to result in significant weight loss in patients.

In clinical trials, people using Byetta® lost an average of 6.6 pounds after thirty weeks and 10.66 pounds after eighty-two

weeks. Byetta®, a synthetic form of a hormone that occurs naturally in the saliva of the Gila monster—a large venomous lizard native to the southwestern United States and Mexico—is injectable
and is usually prescribed along with metformin and a sulfonylurea
or a thiazolidinedione when patients are not achieving glucose targets with pills alone. Byetta® has fewer side effects than many oral
agents; however, most people do experience some nausea in the first
few weeks. "I've had so many patients lose weight on Byetta®," a
diabetes educator told me, "that I would put most of my patients
on it if they weren't afraid of taking injections." Byetta® is only
used for type 2 diabetes.

Symlin® is a synthetic form of a different hormone called
amylin, which is secreted by beta cells after meals to help shut off
one's appetite and level out post-meal glucose peaks. Symylin®
helps patients lose weight by decreasing their appetite and slowing
the rate at which food passes from the stomach to the intestines. A
study published in *Medicine Plus: Journal of Clinical Endocrinology
and Metabolism* in August 2007 showed that among 102 patients
with a body mass index (BMI) of 37.8 (a person with a BMI over
30 is classified as obese) who participated in a sixteen-week trial
using Symlin®, 31 percent lost 5 percent or more of their total
body weight, or roughly eight pounds and one and one-half inches
from their waistlines. What's more, 72 percent of the patients said
their appetite control had improved. Symlin® is an injectable
drug and can be used by anyone who uses insulin.

The skinny about insulin causing weight gain

Insulin causing weight gain is like a sheep in wolf's clothing. For
some people, insulin can produce minor weight gain by enhancing

fat storage and preventing the mobilization of fat into energy. To remedy this, physicians recommend a slight decrease in daily calories and an increase in physical activity to halt weight gain. But usually it's for a different reason that people gain weight using insulin. Well, actually, it's for one of these four different reasons:

1. When blood sugar levels are consistently high, usually before a diagnosis of diabetes or when medication is not controlling diabetes well, glucose builds up in the blood stream. In an effort to get rid of this excess blood sugar, you will urinate frequently. The extra glucose gets excreted, and along with it calories—presto, you lose weight! When you begin using insulin, your blood sugar normalizes, your body stops excreting glucose and calories, and presto, you gain weight! Although it *appears* that insulin is the cause of your weight gain, in fact you are gaining weight because insulin is now allowing your body to absorb the calories it was previously flushing away.

2. Just like some oral medications, insulin can cause hypoglycemia. Thus your appetite increases and you may consume extra calories. Also, hypoglycemia can stimulate a certain panic that causes you to overeat in a rush to get your blood sugar back up. If this happens with any frequency, you'll gain weight. A diabetes educator told me that when patients complain of gaining weight and don't know why, she first asks them whether they're having a lot of lows.

3. If you take an insulin that requires you to eat on a schedule (such as premixed, intermediate, or some longer-acting insulins,) you can't skip meals and may need to eat snacks. This can cause weight gain. If this applies to you, talk to

your health care provider about a possible change in your medication. Often, using a rapid-acting insulin before meals with a long-acting insulin taken once a day, or using an insulin pump, can help you avoid eating extra food.

4. People tend to give themselves more latitude to consume more calories when using insulin: "Oh, I can have dessert. I'll just 'cover' it with some extra insulin." If this becomes a habit, there'll be more of *you* to cover.

Some Teenagers Are Falling Victim to "Diabulimia"

One outgrowth of the fear of gaining weight from using insulin is "diabulimia"—an eating disorder that occurs mostly among teenage girls with type 1 diabetes who skip insulin injections to lose weight. Because high blood sugar causes the body to excrete calories, skipping insulin doses is an easy way to drop a few pounds. This is extremely dangerous behavior, because continuous high blood sugars lead to both short-term harm (such as dehydration, fatigue, and the breakdown of muscle tissue) and the possible earlier onset of long-term diabetic complications (including blindness, kidney disease, and heart disease). As reported by the Juvenile Diabetes Research Foundation, an alarming 30 percent of adolescent type 1 females have skipped or restricted insulin doses in order to lose weight. If you notice this behavior in your child, or in yourself, says Dr. Ann Goebel-Fabbri, a clinical psychologist at the Joslin Diabetes Center who conducts research in this area, try to find both an eating disorder specialist and a diabetes specialist who can help.

MYTH #16

I can't have diabetes because
I have no symptoms.

TRUTH: *Actually*, you can have either type 1 or type 2 diabetes without experiencing, or recognizing, symptoms.

Right now there are approximately six million Americans who have diabetes—both type 1 and type 2—and don't know it. How is this possible? Type 2 diabetes tends to come on slowly, and its symptoms are not always obvious. In the early stage of type 2 diabetes most people experience insulin resistance. It begins as people age, gain weight, and become sedentary, and it slowly worsens over the next several years. It is not unusual to have type 2 diabetes for at least five years before any symptoms become apparent.

It's also easy to attribute many of the symptoms of diabetes to aging. Most people dismiss waking up several times during the night to urinate as a sign of age, but this pattern can be a symptom of diabetes—your body is trying to flush excess sugar out of the blood stream. Although we commonly associate type 2 diabetes with being overweight, when your body flushes sugar away you can also lose weight. Looking back, a friend told me he'd lost significant weight and only thought it was great. He had no idea he had diabetes. Even the most common symptom—extreme thirst—is easy to miss. Dana, a sixteen-year-old girl I interviewed, had no idea her unquenchable thirst was a symptom of diabetes. "I was drinking gallons of water," she told me, "but my parents thought I was thirsty because I was so heavy. Then I went to Florida to visit my grandmother, and I thought I was drinking because of the heat down there. It wasn't until my thirst got so bad I thought I was going to die that we went to the doctor. She said I had diabetes."

Not only do people often overlook a symptom of diabetes, but even large, urban hospitals often don't catch high blood sugar. In 2002, in such a hospital, a chart review of 1,034 adults showed that 13 percent had blood glucose levels greater than 200 mg/dl, yet 36 percent remained undiagnosed at the time of discharge.

At fifty, Terry had no idea he had diabetes until he went to the clinic for a sore back. He had slipped on the ice in a parking lot during a Minnesota winter. While he was sitting on a bench awaiting his X-ray results, the doctor asked whether Terry had any other medical problems. "No, not really, except that I seem to be eating and drinking a lot," he said. Terry's doctor added up what he ate and drank in a day and found that Terry was consuming over 7,000 calories! The doctor took a blood sample with a glucose meter, and Terry's blood sugar was over 500. A fasting blood sugar test confirmed that Terry had diabetes.

You can also have type 1 diabetes, as do more than 2 million Americans, for years before exhibiting the typical symptoms of thirst, frequent urination, and weight loss. Whereas the symptoms appear abruptly in children, the illness can develop more slowly in adolescents and adults, and a diagnosis is often made unexpectedly during a routine exam. Studies conducted by the renowned Joslin

Clinic in Boston show that it can take as long as nine years before symptoms are noticeable in adults.

In my case, the symptoms of my type 1 diabetes presented themselves a few months before my diagnosis, yet I've been told that I was probably losing beta cell function for seven or eight years before that. Oddly, I can pinpoint one specific incident when, had I been aware of the symptoms of diabetes, I would have realized that something was very wrong. It was mid-December and I was riding the bus home on a Christmas break from my university. We stopped at McDonald's midway through the trip, and I brought back onto the bus a large iced tea, a large Coke, a large water, and a small bag of French fries. This followed weeks of gripping the water fountain in my college dormitory every half hour to quench an unquenchable thirst and waking almost nightly at 3 A.M. with excruciating leg cramps. It was the leg cramps that two months later finally got me to the doctor's office for his pronouncement of diabetes.

Common symptoms of type 2 diabetes

The best way to know for sure whether you have diabetes is to be aware of the risk factors and symptoms and to get a fasting blood glucose test and a glucose intolerance test. (For risk factors, refer to Myth #8: So many of my family members have diabetes, I'm certain to get it!) Common symptoms of type 2 diabetes are

- Frequent urination
- Unusual thirst
- Extreme hunger

- Unusual weight loss or gain
- Flu-like feeling, extreme fatigue, weakness, and lack of appetite
- Irritability
- Blurred vision
- Cuts/bruises that are slow to heal, or frequent infections
- Recurring skin, gum, or bladder infections
- Tingling/numbness in the hands/feet
- Acanthosis nigricans—dark patches of skin usually around your neck, elbows, knees, armpits, and groin

Risk factors for type 1 diabetes

- Having a parent or sibling with type 1 diabetes
- Northern European or Mediterranean ancestry
- Drinking cow's milk in infancy
- Having another autoimmune condition, such as Hashimoto's disease, Grave's disease, or celiac disease
- Environmental factors such as stress and exposure to toxins

Common symptoms of type 1 diabetes

- Excessive thirst
- Excessive urination
- Excessive hunger
- Weight loss
- Fatigue
- Blurred vision
- High blood sugar level

- Vaginal yeast infections in girls who haven't yet entered puberty
- Sudden bed-wetting

The most severe symptom of type 1 diabetes is diabetic ketoacidosis. This is a result of the body breaking down fat, instead of carbohydrate, for energy. Ketoacidosis usually occurs only when all the earlier symptoms have gone unnoticed. Symptoms of ketoacidosis are stomach pain, nausea, vomiting, fruity-smelling breath, breathing problems, and a loss of consciousness. Diabetic ketoacidosis is sometimes mistakenly diagnosed as the flu or appendicitis, so be alert if type 1 diabetes is in your family.

If I lose weight and don't require medicine anymore, I'll no longer have diabetes!

TRUTH: *Actually*, the symptoms of type 2 diabetes may go away, but not the condition. If you have type 1 diabetes, then no matter how much weight you lose you will always require insulin, but you may require less.

Once you have diabetes, unless or until a cure is discovered, most physicians consider that you always have diabetes. What may change is how you manage it. Many people with type 2 diabetes may lower their medication requirement and control their blood glucose well enough to actually discontinue medication by losing about 5–10 percent of their body weight and engaging in regular moderate activity such as walking, swimming, or bicycling. This is because weight loss and exercise decrease insulin resistance, helping your body use the insulin it produces more effectively. Still, you aren't considered "cured" of diabetes, because if you regain the weight and become sedentary again, your symptoms of diabetes will return.

If you have type 1 diabetes, you make no or virtually no insulin, and the only treatment is to replace the insulin you no longer make. If you are overweight, you may also be insulin-resistant. If you lose some weight, you may lose some of your insulin resistance. And if you're regularly physically active your insulin sensitivity may increase. Both may cause your insulin requirement to lessen, but neither will change the fact that you will always require some amount of insulin to manage your diabetes.

The benefits of taking less or no medication

Even though you don't "lose" your diabetes, there are several benefits to needing only a lower dose of your medication or none at all.

1. *Reduce or eliminate side effects.* Many medications have side effects. Clinical evidence links some to heart attack, congestive heart failure, or decreased liver and kidney function. Many have not been used or tested long enough for it to be clear what long-term side effects they may have.
2. *Convenience and time saving.* Reducing or eliminating medication gives you greater freedom in eating and more time to do things other than deal with your diabetes.
3. *Cost benefit.* Medications are costly, and the ability to reduce or eliminate your medication can save you a lot of money.
4. *Reduce stress and gain greater peace of mind.* You no longer have to worry about filling prescriptions and performing some of the many diabetes management tasks.

The benefit of using less insulin

If you have type 1 diabetes, even though you will never be able to eliminate your insulin, lowering your dose provides some of the benefits above and possibly greater control. If you have type 2 diabetes and use insulin, you reap the same reward. Dr. Richard Bernstein, author of *The Diabetes Solution: A Complete Guide to*

Achieving Normal Blood Sugars, says that maintaining a very low-carbohydrate diet and being physically active means requiring less insulin. Using less insulin, Dr. Bernstein explains, yields greater predictability and control. It's what he calls the Law of Small Numbers—the less insulin you take, the less variability there is in how much of it actually gets absorbed and used, as well as in how quickly it starts working.

Bernstein cites a study conducted at the University of Minnesota, which demonstrated that when you inject twenty units of insulin, you'll get a whopping 39 percent variation in the amount that gets into your blood stream from one day to the next. When you inject lower doses, particularly under five units, the uncertainty of absorption approaches zero. Dr. Gerald Bernstein confirms that at higher doses, as little as 20–40 percent of the insulin injected gets utilized.

Tip to Make You Tops

Following the Law of Small Numbers, Dr. Richard Bernstein has his patients, who already use small doses of insulin, dose only up to seven units in a single injection. If they take fourteen units, for instance, he has them split the dose into two injections of seven units each. The Law of Small Numbers also provides greater control, because smaller inputs mean smaller errors. Following Bernstein's advice, I changed my diet, which resulted in my using almost a third less insulin. Since then, my blood sugars no longer fluctuate widely, are much easier to keep in range, and are much more predictable.

Weight loss and exercise for becoming symptom- and medication-free

My friend Jon had been living with type 2 diabetes for ten years when he turned fifty, and he'd had it! He was fed up with his 305-pound bulk and the more than eight medications he was taking, so he made a concerted effort to shed pounds—and he did, ninety of them. He cut down on portion sizes, eliminated the fatty and junk foods from the diet he had eaten all his life, and went to the gym five days a week for a cardio and weight-lifting routine. He even worked with a physical trainer one day a week. Now Jon's blood sugars are in the normal range, and he doesn't require or take any blood sugar medication. His other medications have been reduced by more than half.

Jon's Medication Snapshot

Medication	What it treats	Before weight loss	After weight loss
Atenalol	Heart function and blood pressure	50 mg	25 mg
Enalipril	Kidney function	40 mg	10 mg
Lipitor	Cholesterol	20 mg	None; instead, 40 mg of Simvastatin, a weaker version of the generic equivalent Zocor
Glucophage	Blood sugar	1000 mg 2×day	None
Avandia	Blood sugar	4 mg 1×day	None

Bear in mind, while reading Jon's stats, that you don't have to lose an enormous amount of weight or become an uber-exerciser to possibly manage your diabetes without medication. My friend, Terry, was diagnosed with type 2 diabetes at the age of forty-eight. As a teacher at the YMCA, she immediately began taking advantage of her free gym membership, doing a light workout three days a week. She also went to a dietitian and says she actually started eating more—"three squares and three snacks a day"—but healthier, lower-calorie foods. She lost twenty-five pounds over six months and was able to go off her medications.

Another method for becoming symptom- and medication-free

John Dixon, an obesity researcher at Monash University in Melbourne, Australia, believes that gastric lap-band surgery may be a bona fide solution for overweight people with diabetes who can't lose weight because of the medication they're taking. Over the past dozen years, gastric lap-band surgery has rapidly been growing in popularity in the United States as an alternative way to lose weight—and for many, that weight loss translates into better diabetes management, including the abatement of their symptoms and the end of their need for medicines. During gastric lap-band surgery a band is placed around the upper stomach, creating a small pouch through which food can pass, decreasing the amount of food one can consume.

As reported in January 2008 in *Health Day News*, a gastric lap-band study was conducted with diabetes patients classified as obese: those with a BMI between thirty and forty. Half the participants had gastric banding and half attempted to lose weight through diet and exercise. On average, those who had the surgery had lost 20.7 percent of their body weight two years after surgery, and twenty-two of the thirty surgery patients' diabetes had gone into remission. The dieting group had lost only 1.7 percent of their body weight, and just four out of thirty patients' diabetes had gone into remission. The remission, researchers concluded, was attributable to the *amount of weight* the patients lost, not to whether they'd done it through surgery or dieting.

LOOKING THROUGH THE LENS OF . . .
Dr. Richard K. Bernstein, MD

Five Ways to Take Care of Your Diabetes

1. People with diabetes are entitled to the same blood sugars as people without diabetes, and random blood sugars for nondiabetic adults, who are not overweight or pregnant, run around 83 mg/dl (4.6 mmol/l).
2. Based on my research, normal Hgb A1c values for many people run from 4.2 to 4.6 percent—not as wide a range as 4 to 6 percent, as some organizations say.
3. The major dietary cause of high blood sugars, coronary disease, and obesity is carbohydrates, not fats. Lessen your carbohydrates for better blood glucose control.
4. Injections and finger sticks are truly painless when properly performed. Find out how.
5. The major cause of amputations in people with diabetes is a patient attempting to remove a callus from his or her foot. Only have a qualified foot specialist tend to your feet.

MYTH #18

There's nothing new for treating type 2 diabetes.

TRUTH: *Actually,* a lot is new, including surgical procedures and innovative drugs.

This explanation is a little longer than some, precisely because so much is new in diabetes treatment and care. Researchers have a greater understanding of the interplay between hormones and blood sugar control, and this insight has given rise to new procedures. Increasing awareness of the importance of patient responsibility has prompted new models for behavior modification. New diabetes drugs not only don't put weight on you, they actually help you lose it, and surgery is being viewed by some as a cure.

Gastric bypass surgery involves sectioning off a small pouch from the upper part of the stomach and attaching it to the lower part of the small intestine, leaving only a small area of the stomach to hold food. This approach was once recommended only for morbidly obese people facing severe health threats, but today it is being performed on more than 140,000 overweight people in the United States each year, a large number of whom have type 2 diabetes. And it's revealing startling results—blood sugar levels return to normal even before any weight loss. When asked in an April 2008 *60 Minutes* interview whether he considered gastric bypass surgery a cure for diabetes, Dr. Neil Hutcher, a gastrointestinal surgeon in Richmond, Virginia, who has performed more than 3,000 bypass surgeries, replied, "I think my patients are cured. They go home on no medication, and I've followed them now for ten and fifteen years and see no evidence of recurrence."

The CBS report said studies confirm that about 80 percent of people with type 2 diabetes who've had gastric bypass surgery go into complete remission within days of their operation. Dr. David Cummings, appetite expert and professor of medicine at the University of Washington, confirmed the remission rate at 84 percent, saying, "A third of patients walk out of the hospital three days after their surgery completely off their diabetes medications, and most of the others shed their diabetes medications within a few weeks."

In 2003 Dr. Philip Schauer, MD, director of the Bariatric Metabolic Institute at the Cleveland Clinic in Cleveland, Ohio, and president of the American Society for Bariatric Surgery (ASBS), was one of the first to show that after bariatric surgery, patients' blood sugars returned to normal before any significant weight loss. "Part of this is explained by what bariatric surgery does to the gastrointestinal tract," said Dr. Schauer. "We now know that there is an alteration of the gut (gastrointestinal) hormones which affect both insulin production and utilization." Scientists are discovering that certain of these gut hormones, called incretins, affect glycemic control far more dramatically than once was thought.

Dr. Francesco Rubino, a pioneering authority in gastrointestinal metabolic surgery and chief of gastrointestinal metabolic surgery at New York Presbyterian/Weill Cornell, is advancing "diabetes surgery" as an entirely new field, one in which gastrointestinal operations can be performed to directly treat diabetes, not just obesity. Dr. Rubino's "diabetes surgery" has been performed on obese patients at several centers worldwide, and clinical trials have begun on diabetes patients who are not obese.

Tip to Make You Tops

Performing research on diabetic rats, Dr. Francesco Rubino saw that when he disconnected the top of the small intestine (duodenum) from the stomach, the rats' diabetes disappeared. Then he reversed the operation and the diabetes returned. By merely blocking food from traveling through the duodenum, Rubino sent rats with diabetes into remission, clear evidence that blood sugar control is connected to gut hormones and can be normalized independent of weight loss.

At the 68th ADA Scientific Conference, Dr. Christopher Sorli of the Billings Clinic in Billings, Montana, reported that a sleeve placed inside sixteen patients with type 2 diabetes to prevent food from going through their duodenums, improved glycemic control as early as one week after the implant, independent of weight loss. Most patients who received the sleeve were also able to stop their diabetes medication. The sleeve is less invasive than gastric bypass surgery yet has similar results.

Laparoscopic gastric banding is another surgical procedure that helps promote weight loss and, as a result, may free patients from medication. During gastric banding an adjustable band is placed around the upper portion of the stomach, sectioning off only a small pouch to hold food. With this procedure the resolution of diabetes goes hand in hand with the resolution of body weight, says Dr. David Cummings. Banding does not "cure" diabetes as does gastric bypass, which affects the hormones responsible for blood sugar metabolism. Yet banding was reported to be a more effective treatment for diabetes than the best current medical care with existing medicines, diet, and exercise.

New advancements for improved blood sugar control

One of the most recent innovations in glucose control is the continuous glucose monitor (CGM). CGMs are tiny wire sensors that go under the skin and send information about glucose levels via a radio transmitter to a pager-sized receiver; they relay your glucose level every few minutes, thus enabling you to see trends and patterns. This helps wearers respond almost immediately to rising or dropping blood sugars. Most people who use CGMs wear an insulin pump, but a pump is not required to use a CGM.

Another breakthrough on the horizon is the artificial pancreas now in clinical trials. An artificial pancreas involves a continuous glucose monitor, an insulin pump, and a control system, all working together to automatically sense and dispense the correct amount of insulin—without patient administration. Researchers project that in only a few years, the artificial pancreas will be a viable alternative to insulin pumps and multiple daily injections of insulin for patients.

Innovative delivery devices and oral insulin

Inhalable insulin was short-lived when, in 2006, Pfizer released the most revolutionary delivery option for insulin since its discovery, an inhalable insulin called Exubera. Unfortunately, the device was unwieldy, similar to the size of a can of tennis balls, and doctors were concerned about long-term lung function. Pfizer abandoned the product, and two other pharmaceutical companies that were conducting trials with inhalable insulin put on the brakes. However, in a *New York Times* November 2007 report titled "Betting an Estate on Inhaled Insulin," entrepreneur Alfred E. Mann is so certain he can succeed with an inhalable insulin that he's putting $1 billion of his own money into redeveloping it. Mr. Mann says his insulin device will be slightly larger than a cell phone and has not so far caused lung problems, although more testing is needed.

Several other insulin-delivery devices are in the prototype stage, including an insulin patch that administers insulin through the skin (like a nicotine patch), insulin nasal and cheek sprays, and what's been a long-awaited dream, insulin in a pill—which is now in clinical trials with patients who have type 2 diabetes. Thus far the results show early success, with a reduction in blood glucose levels and an increase in insulin levels.

A new class of diabetes drugs

"Until 1995, there had been no substantial advance in drug management of diabetes since the 1950s," said John Buse, an endocrinologist at the University of North Carolina at Chapel Hill and president of the American Diabetes Association. In the last few years, however, several new diabetes medications have come to market.

A very recent class of drugs, incretin mimetics (drugs that mimic the effect of certain gut hormones), improve the body's ability to manage glucose levels by stimulating insulin secretion when food is eaten, slowing stomach emptying, and inhibiting the liver from secreting glucagon, a hormone involved in carbohydrate metabolism. These drugs have been proved useful in weight loss, and they improve blood sugar control before and after meals. An increasing number of endocrinologists believe that post-meal blood sugar control is more significant than was previously thought as a way to prevent diabetic complications.

Tip to Make You Tops

James, a fifty-nine-year-old photographer who had type 2 diabetes for nine years, felt utterly defeated trying to keep his blood sugars near, let alone in, target range. His mother and older brother had died of diabetic complications, and his other brother, who also had type 2 diabetes, was on kidney dialysis. However, a year after I met James he was taking Byetta®, and his blood sugars were in target range most of the time. He'd lost several pounds and had an entirely different outlook on life.

Byetta® is one such drug. In trials, more than four times as many patients using Byetta® along with other medications reached the ADA's recommended A1C level of less than 7 percent, and a majority of patients lost an average of eight pounds in thirty weeks.

Symlin®, another new medication, replaces the hormone amylin, which is produced by beta cells and lost as beta cells degrade. Symlin® suppresses the release of glucagon from the liver, flattening post-meal blood sugars, which researchers now know is important to help prevent diabetes complications and slows down the absorption of carbohydrates, promoting satiety and weight loss.

Tip to Make You Tops

Because Byetta® and Symlin® slow stomach emptying, they are not recommended for patients with gastroparesis, who already experience slow emptying of the stomach. Significant slow stomach emptying makes timing insulin injections extremely difficult.

Januvia® is a pill that reduces the amount of glucose made by the liver and stimulates the release of insulin only when there are available carbohydrates, decreasing the incidence of hypoglycemia. Januvia® is well tolerated by most patients and causes neither weight loss nor weight gain.

Insulin has been around since 1921, but in the last few years newer types of insulin have been developed that help control blood sugar more effectively thanks to their quicker onset, less pronounced peak, and quick degradation. (For more information, refer to Myth #21: If I take insulin, I must eat snacks during the day and at bedtime.)

Additional advances in better management

Recent studies indicate that regardless of new devices, medicines, and knowledge, patients are not likely to have better outcomes if they fail to adopt healthier behaviors. So diabetes education is shifting from telling patients what to do to partnering with and coaching patients to make manageable changes in their diet, exercise, and stress management. Modifying behaviors creates sustainability over the long haul.

Peer mentoring is also emerging in diabetes care to help fill the gap between the decreasing number of endocrinologists and diabetes educators and the increasing number of patients. Patient Mentor Institute (PMI) trains mentors and offers free peer-mentoring programs to diabetes educators. To learn more, contact PMI through its Web site: http://patientmentor.org or call: 866-741-7047. The American Academy of Family Physicians Foundation, in partnership with the American Association of Diabetes Educators and the American Academy of Family Physicians, is developing a global peer-to-peer mentoring program called Peers for Progress. You can learn more on its Web site: www.peersforprogress.org.

MYTH #19

If I'm sick (such as with a cold or flu) and barely eat, I shouldn't take my diabetes medicine.

TRUTH: *Actually*, you probably should. Your blood sugar is likely to rise from the physical stress of being sick, even though you are not eating.

It might seem that if you're not eating much because you're sick, you should take less medication or none at all, but just the opposite is likely to be true. Illness, infection, and injury all create stress on your body. Stress hormones are then released, causing your liver to send extra glucose into your blood stream to give your body extra energy to fight the illness. That means your blood sugar will probably go up. So even if you're barely eating because you're too fatigued, or feel nauseated, or even are vomiting, you'll probably need your usual amount of medicine or possibly more. (Note: Metformin may need to be temporarily discontinued if you have the flu or are having difficulty keeping fluids down. Check with your health care provider.)

If you take insulin it seems counterintuitive to take more while you're eating less, but for most people, including myself, that's just what you need to do. But be aware that not every sniffle will affect your blood sugar; the only way to know whether it has done so is to test your blood sugar every few hours. If it's high, call your health care provider, or, if you're adept at adjusting your insulin, increase your dose by one or two units to see whether this returns your blood sugar to target range. If you don't use insulin and need to reduce your blood sugar level, eat a little less carbohydrates or take a short walk if you're feeling well enough. If your blood sugar goes way up and won't come down, you may need to take insulin temporarily. Keeping your blood sugars within or as close to your target range as possible will help you both feel better and heal faster.

Tip to Make You Tops

My friend Ann, who has type 2 diabetes and uses short- and long-acting insulin, has worked out a sick-day plan with her doctor. Ann (1) checks her blood sugar eight times a day instead of her normal four or five, especially an hour and a half after meals, (2) keeps her carbohydrate intake up with juice, hot tea with honey, soup and crackers, yogurt, applesauce, and ice cream, and (3) uses sugar-free medications, such as cough syrup and throat lozenges.

Choosing easy-to-digest foods when you're sick

Carbohydrates are essential while you're ill, because they provide much-needed energy and speed healing. If eating is a problem because you have no appetite or a high fever, you still need to try to eat your usual amount of carbohydrates. All of the following foods are easy to digest and contain 15–20 grams of carbohydrate, which is equivalent to one carbohydrate exchange.

- ½ cup regular soda (not diet)
- ½ cup fruit juice

- ½ cup ice cream
- ¼ cup sherbet
- ½ cup cooked cereal
- 1 slice toast
- 1 cup soup
- 6 saltine crackers
- 3 graham crackers
- ½ cup regular gelatin (not sugar-free)
- 1 Popsicle or fruit juice bar

Tip to Make You Tops

Check the total carbohydrates in sports drinks before you drink them. Many contain a large amount which may make your blood sugar rise too high.

Recognizing and managing dehydration

In addition to keeping your carbohydrate intake when you're sick similar to what it is when you're not sick, it's important not to get dehydrated. Dehydration is a loss of body fluids that contain vital minerals, such as sodium and potassium, and is usually caused by vomiting, diarrhea, or not eating or drinking enough. Dehydration can put a strain on your cardiovascular system, affecting your heart, kidneys, and brain. Its warning signs include thirst, headache, dizziness, fatigue, weakness, irritability, heat flush, vomiting, nausea, and muscle cramps. Dehydration may also rob your body of its ability to rid your blood stream of extra sugar.

To avoid dehydration, sip water and, if you like, sugar-free or caffeine-free liquids throughout the day. One diabetes educator advises her patients to take a few sips of liquid during each commercial break if watching TV. If you're feeling well enough, eating fresh fruits and vegetables will also replenish water in your system. Ingesting fluids that contain sodium, such as broth, tomato juice, and sports drinks, is also important to help retain fluid and replenish mineral loss.

Because it can be harder to keep your blood sugar in target range when you're sick, work out a plan with your diabetes educator or health care provider so that you know, before you get sick, what to do when the need arises. Make sure your sick-day plan includes how often you should measure your blood sugar, your target blood sugar range, how to handle your medicine, what you should eat and drink, which foods or beverages you should avoid, and what specific symptoms should prompt a call to your doctor.

MYTH #20

If my diabetes is under control, there's no need to see my doctor.

TRUTH: *Actually,* because you may not notice any symptoms at the beginning of many diabetic complications, seeing your doctor regularly is important both to prevent complications and to detect them early.

Keeping your blood sugar as close to normal as you safely can is hands down the best way to reduce your risk of diabetic complications. Yet, it's not a guarantee. For some people, even well-controlled diabetes may result in some complications, and people with type 1 diabetes are susceptible to complications because of the length of time they have diabetes and the impossibility of keeping blood sugars perfectly controlled all the time. (Still, that's no reason not to do your best to manage your diabetes.) Given this, however, and the fact that many complications begin with no noticeable symptoms, it's important to see your doctor on a regular basis and get screened for complications at least annually.

Hypertension (high blood pressure) is referred to as the "silent killer" because you aren't likely to know you have it without a blood pressure check. There are no noticeable symptoms for high cholesterol or high triglycerides. Nor will you feel anything at the early stages of kidney disease. You may notice no change in your vision even if you have early stages of diabetic retinopathy, or you may hear, as I did five years ago from my ophthalmologist, that you have a slow-growing cataract. Catching my cataract early and having my ophthalmologist keep an eye on it (no pun intended), will enable us to take care of it as soon as necessary and avoid a serious problem.

Peripheral neuropathy, damage to the nerves, causes many people to lose sensation in their feet. They can get cuts, burns, skin cracks, or blisters, or even step on a nail, and not know it! If any of these conditions is not treated early, the tissue and bones of the feet can get infected and cause a foot ulcer, an extremely serious condition. Foot ulcers often precede a lower-extremity amputation.

Still in his forties, Bob got diabetes five years ago and wasn't taking care of it. When Bob was first diagnosed, his doctor put him on an oral medication, and when the prescription ran out Bob never refilled it. He hadn't seen his doctor since. Luckily for Bob, his wife finally got him back to the doctor, who told him he saw some early damage to his eyes. Bob realized that the time for fooling around was over and made appointments with an ophthalmologist and cardiologist for the following week. He's now back on his medication.

Prescription for lowering the odds of complications

If you take oral medications or are managing your diabetes with diet and exercise alone, you should see your doctor every four to six months. If you take insulin, the general recommendation is to see your doctor every three to four months. Of course, this schedule also depends on your individual needs—more frequent visits may be necessary if your blood sugar is not well controlled, if you feel unwell, or if you have complications that are getting worse. The importance of regular doctor visits, foot and eye examinations, and blood and urine tests can't be overstated: Diabetes affects all your vital organs as well as your micro- and macrovascular systems, including your brain, heart, kidney, eyes, and feet, and your gastric, nerve, and circulatory systems.

The tests listed below are recommended for everyone with diabetes. Although the list may seem daunting, several of these tests can be performed from a single blood draw. Discuss with your health care provider how often you should have these tests, what your test results mean, and (if need be) what steps you should take to improve your test results. Remember: It's your body, your health, and your future you're safeguarding.

Tip to Make You Tops

To keep track of when it's time to get your tests, write them down on a calendar and group them around a special event such as your birthday.

---

1. Hemoglobin A1c

The A1C test reflects your average blood glucose level over the entire day—before and after meals, between meals, while sleeping etc.—and over the past two to three months. This test gives the best indication of how well your blood sugars are being managed. Blood for this test is drawn either in a doctor's office or in a laboratory. The ADA recommends that people with diabetes have an A1C of less than 7 percent, and the American Association of Clinical Endocrinologists (AACE) advises an A1C of less than 6.5 percent. If your A1C is consistently within your target range, you might have this test just twice a year. If you have trouble keeping your blood sugar within target range or if you start a new diabetes medication, you should have this test four times a year. [The ADA's 2009 Standards of Care advises clinicians to use the eAG, a mathematical formula that translates A1C values into the same units you see on your glucometer.] Don't forget, however, that the A1C and eAG are average values; an A1C of 7 percent, the equivalent to an eAG of about 150 mg/dl (8.3 mmol/l), could mean that your blood glucose is 50 mg/dl (2.7 mmol/l) half the time and 250 mg/dl (13.8 mg/dl) the other half.

2. Lipids test—Checks HDL, LDL, and triglycerides

This test measures the level of lipids (fats) in your blood, including low-density lipoprotein (LDL), aka "bad cholesterol"; high-density lipoprotein (HDL), aka "good cholesterol," which protects against heart disease; and triglycerides, unused calories stored as fat. High levels of triglycerides increase your risk of heart disease. It is recommended to get a lipids test yearly, and more often if you're taking lipid-lowering medication (statins). Optimal levels for your LDL, HDL, and triglycerides are

- LDL lower than 100 mg/dl; lower than 70 if underlying heart disease
- HDL higher than 50 mg/dl for women and higher than 40 mg/dl for men
- Triglycerides lower than 150 mg/dl

3. Blood pressure—Routine cuff test

It's estimated that two out of three people with type 2 diabetes have high blood pressure, and the condition is particularly common among African Americans. Blood pressure should be taken at every visit to your health care provider. In this simple procedure, a rubber cuff is wrapped around your upper arm and inflated. As the air releases from the cuff, a measuring instrument indicates the systolic pressure, the pressure of your blood flow when your heart beats (the first number in 130/80 mm/Hg) and the diastolic pressure, the pressure between heartbeats (the second number in the formula). High blood pressure strains the heart and damages blood vessels. The American Diabetes Association recommends a target blood pressure of less than 130/80 mm/Hg.

Tip to Make You Tops

Treatment options for high blood pressure include lifestyle changes such as lowering your sodium and alcohol intake, maintaining a healthy weight, engaging in regular exercise, and not smoking. Your health care provider may also recommend medications such as angiotensin receptor blockers (ARBs) and angiotensin-converting enzyme (ACE) inhibitors. ARBs help lower blood pressure, reduce fluid retention, and control heart failure. ACE inhibitors help widen blood vessels, which lowers blood pressure and takes strain off the heart.

---

4. Microalbumin test

This test assesses the health of your kidneys by screening for protein in your urine: If your kidneys become damaged, protein that should remain in your blood leaks into your urine. This test requires providing a sample of urine at your doctor's office or a laboratory. A normal microalbumin level is less than 30 mg. Above 30 mg indicates early-stage kidney disease, and above 300 mg indicates advanced kidney disease. It's recommended that you have this test annually, but if your microalbumin levels are high, you may be advised to have it more often. ACE inhibitors and ARBs have proved effective in slowing the progression of kidney disease. Your doctor may also recommend making certain changes to your diet, such as decreasing the amount of protein you eat.

5. Serum creatinine and BUN (blood urea nitrogen) tests

These tests measure how effectively your kidneys are filtering small molecules out of your blood. The normal range for creatinine in women is 0.7 to 1.2 mg/dl (62 to 106 umol/l) and for men, 0.9 to 1.4 mg/dl (80 to 106 umol/l). Normal values for the BUN test are 10 to 20 mg/dl (3.6 to 7.1 mmol/l). These tests are typically done once a year.

6. Dilated eye exam

An optometrist or ophthalmologist should perform a dilated eye exam annually. This entails having a few drops of liquid placed in your eyes so that the specialist can see the back of your eye, where damage to the small blood vessels can occur. Eye damage can occur with no noticeable disturbance to your vision. If the condition is caught early, laser therapy can correct damage already done or stop it from progressing.

LOOKING THROUGH THE LENS OF . . .
Francine Ratner Kaufman, Pediatric Endocrinologist

Five Ways to Take Care of Your Diabetes

1. Let your friends and co-workers know you have diabetes. If you let them know that you are in control of your diabetes and that diabetes management tasks are part of your regular routine, they will view those tasks as just as natural as breathing and eating.

2. Don't try to do it all alone. It takes a support system—your spouse, your children, your parents, your friends—to keep you motivated and on the right track.

3. Be prepared for an emergency. Never leave home without supplies, and have them wherever you visit frequently.

4. Know your numbers, and keep copies of your medical visits and labs. The changing health care environment makes it important for you to have everything that is critical to your health in your own files, as well as in those of your doctors. The labs are yours; keep the results in a notebook or in your computer, so that you maximally participate in your diabetes care.

5. Find the right team. Your doctors, nurses, and dietitians are on your journey with you. You are at the helm. They are there to help steer, to advise, and to plan with you, but you are the one ultimately in charge.

7. Foot exam

You should check your feet daily and remind your doctor to check your feet at every visit. You may also get care from a foot specialist such as a podiatrist. During a foot exam, a specialist checks your foot structure, joint mobility, gait, and balance, in addition to the skin between your toes and on the ball of your foot and the pulse in your feet. Don't overlook your feet. High blood sugars make you particularly vulnerable to serious foot problems that you may not feel.

MYTH #21

If I take insulin, I must eat snacks during the day and at bedtime.

TRUTH: *Actually*, newer rapid-acting insulins and long-acting insulins don't require consistent snacking.

Older insulins such as Regular®, NPH®, Humulin L Lente®, and Humulin U Ultralente®, because of their pronounced peaks and duration in the body, require that you eat snacks in order to prevent hypoglycemia. Regular® peaks between two and four hours after injecting and stays in your system for six to eight hours. That means it's still lowering your blood glucose long after your meal has stopped raising it. NPH® peaks about six hours after injecting and leaves your system in about sixteen, Lente® peaks nearly eight to nine hours after injecting and exits in about twenty, and Ultralente® peaks about twelve hours after injecting and lasts almost twenty-four hours total. If you're using one of these insulins, you need to eat regularly timed snacks.

However, today's long-acting insulins (Lantus® and Levemir®) and rapid-acting mealtime insulins (Humalog®, Novolog®, and Apidra®), which came to market three to ten years ago, do not require eating snacks, and most patients on these insulins don't do so. Of course, based on how these insulins affect you and your individual diabetes goals, your treatment plan may call for a snack at a particular time of day.

Rapid-acting insulins:
Humalog®, Novolog®, and Apidra®

These insulins are called "bolus" insulins and are used specifically to cover the carbohydrates in meals and snacks. Their greatest advantage is how quickly they go to work and how quickly they exit the body. They begin working between five and fifteen minutes after injecting, peak in one to one and a half hours, and clear out of the body within three to four hours. The faster action and shorter duration of these insulins enable them to better match the "action time" of your meals; they generally reach their peak when your blood glucose is at its highest, so they're lowering your blood sugar at the same time food is raising it. Between three and four hours later, when any of these bolus insulins is leaving your system, your blood sugar is near to its starting point.

Because the composition of your meal determines how quickly your blood sugar will rise, rapid-acting insulins allow you to achieve better pre- and post-meal blood sugar control. Foods that have a high glycemic index (GI), those that break down rapidly and release glucose quickly into the bloodstream, such as cold cereals, juice, and soda, are easier to cover with rapid-acting insulins. When eating low-GI carbohydrates, those that digest slowly, such as brown rice or a bean burrito or eating a meal with considerable fat in it, which slows the rise of blood sugar, you can best match your blood sugar's rise by injecting during or after your meal or by taking half your dose before the meal and half your dose an hour or two after eating. To manage the "dawn phenomenon" (a condition marked by a significant and rapid rise in early-morning blood glucose that many insulin-dependent patients experience), I often take one-third of my breakfast bolus upon waking to blunt the rise and the other two-thirds just before or during my meal (steel cut oatmeal, a low-GI food.) These are general guidelines. Talk to your health care provider to work out your personal plan.

Tip to Make You Tops

When I switched from Humalog® to Apidra®, I had to switch my injection from before my meal to after—Apidra® worked much faster for me. It was a great advantage to inject after my meal: With no guesswork about what, exactly, I'd end up eating, I could match my insulin more precisely. If you're starting on a rapid-acting insulin, test your blood sugar often—before a meal, two hours after a meal, and before you go to sleep—to determine how fast it works in your body.

Long-acting insulins: Lantus® and Levemir®

Lantus® and Levemir® are called "basal" insulins. They last between sixteen and twenty-four hours, are generally taken once or twice a day, and mimic a normally functioning pancreas by continuously delivering small amounts of insulin to keep blood sugar at normal levels between meals. These insulins are nearly peakless, offering the benefit of reduced hypoglycemic events with their flatter action. If you use Lantus® or Levemir®, your health care provider will adjust your dose so that you don't need to snack. However, if you also take an oral medication that can cause hypoglycemia, you may need a bedtime snack.

If you are on large doses of basal insulin (70–100 units or more in one injection), it may work more effectively if you split your dose into two injections taken at the same time. For instance, you might take 35–50 units in each of two separate injections. Because long-acting insulins vary in duration from about nineteen to twenty-four hours, your doctor may also prescribe that you use them once or twice a day. When my friend Ruth switched from using Lantus® once a day to using it twice a day, her blood sugar control improved dramatically.

Tip to Make You Tops

Before Lantus® came to market, I used Humulin L®, a long-acting insulin, and no matter how carefully I timed my snacks, its peaking action woke me almost nightly at 3 A.M., when I'd find myself soaked through my pajamas and babbling in a semi-coherent low-blood-sugar stupor. My husband may miss playing Prince Valiant by bringing me glucose tablets, but I have not awakened in the middle of the night with low blood sugar since starting Lantus® four years ago.

I've heard for thirty years that there's going to be a cure for type 1 diabetes, but nothing's changed.

TRUTH: *Actually,* some consider islet cell transplantation a cure, and other advances made over the last five to ten years have vastly improved living with type 1 diabetes.

I got type 1 diabetes thirty-seven years ago and every few years I heard, "In ten years there'll be a cure," but for the first twenty years of my diabetes-life, nothing much seemed to happen. Today, however, advances in research and technology have led to watershed developments. On the biological front, some physicians and patients consider islet cell transplantation a cure, and regeneration, the replenishing of insulin-producing beta cells, is a hotbed of dynamic and aggressive research. The advent of new technologies has yielded revolutionary devices such as the continuous glucose monitor, smart and tubeless insulin pumps, small feature-packed meters, even an electronic lancing device. And one of the most highly anticipated breakthroughs, an artificial pancreas, is now in clinical trials. More has changed in the last several years than in the past thirty years combined.

Scientific Research Accelerates on Three Fronts

The biological front

The Diabetes Research Institute (DRI), a recognized world leader in cure-focused diabetes research, performed its first islet cell transplant in 1990. Nine years later, in Edmonton, Canada, scientists performed islet transplants on seven patients, proving to the medical community that islet transplantation *can* work. The procedure is known as the Edmonton Protocol. As reported by the Mayo Clinic in a study published in 2006, more than 40 percent of thirty-six islet cell transplant recipients were off insulin within one year of the transplant. Two years later, however, less than 14 percent of recipients remained insulin-free. Even so, scientists remain enormously hopeful that islet cell transplantation *will* work.

"Not since the polio vaccine was developed in the 1950s have medical researchers been as enthusiastic about the possible cure of another of the world's most devastating diseases as they are now," wrote Jaron Terry in Ohio State University Medical Center's 2007 article, "Islet Cell Transplant: Is This the Cure for Type 1 Diabetes?" OSUMC is one of a select group of medical centers across North America approved to process pancreatic islet cells for human transplant.

"Islet cell transplantation is a wonderful experiment but not a clinical solution for most patients," says Dr. Fred Levine, adjunct professor at The Burnham Institute for Medical Research in California. However, it provides a perfect platform for regeneration research. Regeneration is the growth, replication, and replenishment of insulin-producing beta cells. The key (and the trick) is getting the cells to work in the body and not be rejected. The fantasy, says

---

Tip to Make You Tops

Islet cell transplantation extracts islets, or clusters of cells that contain beta cells, from a donor pancreas and infuses them into a recipient's liver. (Islet cells do well in the liver, and it's difficult to get them into the pancreas because of where it is situated in the body.) Only people with type 1 diabetes who have severe complications such as "hypoglycemic unawareness" (a condition wherein you don't get the warning signals of low blood sugar) and patients who can't effectively manage their diabetes with insulin are candidates.

In New York City in 2007, I interviewed a young woman named Amy who, because of her severe hypoglycemic unawareness, had had two islet cell transplants, the first having failed after only a few months. Amy had gotten type 1 at the age of eleven, about twenty years earlier, and since college she had nearly fallen into a coma from countless episodes of hypoglycemic unawareness. It would happen walking to work, driving a car, while in a meeting, lying in bed. After her second transplant Amy was insulin-free for eighteen months. "I considered myself cured, absolutely," she said, and although she now has to take a small amount of insulin, her warning symptoms of hypoglycemia have returned. "Since the islet cell transplant, my husband has not had to wake me up in the middle of the night to see if I'm still alive. Before, he used to do that every single night."

Dr. Levine, is that we can hand people two pills: one causes beta cells to form, and the other causes the body not to reject them. The fantasy may not be all that far-off: Scientists at Edinburgh University recently took the first step toward purifying new pancreas cells, and the DRI has had early success getting liver cells to function as islet cells. Clinical human trials are growing beta cells both inside and outside of the human body, and researchers are currently working to turn off the immune system so it won't destroy new pancreatic cells, and they are studying Byetta® (a glucose-lowering injectable for people with type 2 diabetes) as a possible regenerator of beta cells.

More than a dozen different programs to preserve and regenerate pancreatic islet cells are occurring internationally, and regeneration is the Juvenile Diabetes Research Foundation's (JDRF) fastest-growing area of supported research. (The JDRF is the leading funder of type 1 diabetes research worldwide.) In addition, technology is providing new breakthroughs in regeneration research, as with magnetic resonance imaging (MRI), which now enables scientists to noninvasively locate, count, and track beta cells.

The technology front

The ultimate technological breakthrough is the artificial pancreas, and researchers believe they are a few short years away from patients using this device. The artificial pancreas, also known as a mechanical pancreas, has three components: a continuous glucose monitor to give a constant accurate reading of blood sugar, an insulin pump to automatically dispense the appropriate amount of insulin, and a control system to ensure that the exact measure of insulin is dispensed as needed. All three will work in concert to mimic the way the pancreas works.

Dr. Roman Hovorka at the University of Cambridge has been testing devices in patients, as has the DRI, which is now addressing safety issues to prevent malfunctions and operator failures. Dr. Aaron Kowalski of the JDRF is working closely with Dr. Hovorka and his team to speed funds to artificial pancreas study teams. U.S.

Food and Drug Administration regulators are also working to design studies that will lead to quicker review. The hope is that the first generation of devices will be out by the spring of 2009.

Additional advances in management devices are already available. They include

- The Omnipod—A tubeless pump consisting of a pod-like shell that contains an insulin reservoir and a wireless remote to program the pod's delivery of insulin.
- Continuous glucose monitor (CGM)—See Myth #18 for details. Medtronic's wireless technology allows its CGM to transmit glucose readings directly to its pump.
- Animas's OneTouch® Ping Glucose Management System—The first insulin pump that wirelessly communicates with a blood glucose meter, providing greater convenience and flexibility.
- The Intuity Meter—Slated to be available in 2009, it tests blood sugar with no test strips. You put your finger over a hole at the bottom of the meter, whereupon it pricks your finger and, in seconds, reads your blood sugar.
- The Pelikan Sun—A nearly painless lancing device, battery-operated with thirty depth settings. It was initially developed to protect the sensitive skin of children.

The delivery front

Delivering insulin in a pill was long just a dream, because digestive juices in the mouth degrade insulin, destroying its efficacy. Today, however, Oramed, an Israeli biotechnology company, is conducting clinical trials for oral insulin. Although the current trials are with people who have type 2 diabetes, researchers believe their findings will ultimately benefit those with type 1 diabetes as well. Dr. Miriam Kidron, chief medical officer of Oramed, says the company has technologically overcome the problem of insulin being destroyed by the gastrointestinal tract, and the results of the trial thus far show a reduction in blood glucose levels and an increase in insulin levels.

Dr. Gerald Bernstein, vice president of Medical Affairs with Generex Biotechnology, is enthusiastic about a product that Generex is developing. Insulin will be absorbed through the lining of the inner mouth, leaving no deposit in the lungs. Because I take multiple daily injections, needless to say I share Dr. Bernstein's enthusiasm. Insulin patch technology and, strange as it sounds, an insulin suppository are also being explored.

Although I may not see a cure in my lifetime, I am genuinely excited about the recent advances in diabetes research, procedures, tools, and medicines. One of the latest is the development of a "smart insulin," part of an operating system whereby when the body detects a spike in glucose, it will release an appropriate amount of insulin from a reservoir of once-daily-injected insulin, to keep blood sugar level. All these advances give me hope that my life can be just as long, productive, and satisfying as anyone else's. And that I may even live long enough to eat my words and actually see a cure.

Women with diabetes shouldn't get pregnant.

TRUTH: *Actually*, this mantra, still told to thousands of women today, is no longer true.

I was eighteen years old when I was diagnosed with type 1 diabetes; one minute I was a freshman in college, and the next I was lying in a hospital bed with my life spinning off its axis. While learning how to give myself injections, which I would have to do for the rest of my life, and hearing I might go blind, I was also told I could never have children. That was thirty-seven years ago. That edict, "You can't have children," is no longer true. Thanks to today's knowledge and technologies, women with both type 1 and type 2 diabetes can indeed have children. However, a woman's diabetes has to be in good control before and throughout her pregnancy, to safeguard her health and the health of her baby.

The key to a healthy pregnancy is good blood sugar control and pre-pregnancy planning. Experts recommend that a woman work with her obstetrician and an endocrinologist three to six months prior to conception so that her blood sugar, blood pressure, cholesterol levels, and heart and vascular health are such that it is safe for her to become pregnant.

Safeguarding your health and that of your baby before pregnancy

A fetus's heart, brain, nervous system, and other organs begin forming during the first five weeks of pregnancy, usually before a woman even knows she is pregnant. This early stage of pregnancy poses risks, including birth defects and spontaneous abortion, says Dr. Lois Jovanovič, MD, professor of medicine and chief scientific officer at the Sansum Diabetes Research Institute. That is why it's critical to be in good health before you conceive. If a woman is already in control of her blood sugar at the time of conception, birth defects are much less likely to happen. If you are considering becoming pregnant, make sure the following vitals are in good order:

Weight—Try to reach a healthy weight before conceiving. Women who are overweight are at increased risk for gestational diabetes, hypertensive disorders of pregnancy, cesarean deliveries, and anesthetic and postoperative complications.

Eyes—Pregnancy can irritate diabetic eye disease (retinopathy). Have an exam with an ophthalmologist who is an expert in retinopathy.

Heart—Heart disease affects women with diabetes at much higher rates and puts you at risk for pregnancy-related complications such as strokes and heart disease. The recommendations for heart disease screening include

- A pre-pregnancy evaluation by your physician for risk of heart disease.
- A resting electrocardiogram (ECG) test before or during pregnancy if you are older than thirty-five.

- Treat risk factors such as high blood pressure, elevated lipids, and smoking.
- Eat two oily, low-mercury fish meals per week or take fish oil capsules.

Blood pressure—High blood pressure (BP) significantly adds to a pregnancy's risks, so have your BP measured at every visit. If your blood pressure is higher than 130/80 mmHg, and that reading is confirmed by a second test on a separate day, your blood pressure should be treated during pregnancy with medication to help you achieve a BP of 110–129 mmHg over 65–79 mmHg.

Tip to Make You Tops

Dr. Lois Jovanovič advises that ACE inhibitors and ARBs not be taken during pregnancy, and that if you're taking them now, you should stop when pregnancy is anticipated. Check with your physician.

Safeguard your health and that of your baby during pregnancy

Tight control of blood sugar during pregnancy is the most effective way to guard against birth defects that originate during the first weeks of gestation. These include damage to the baby's heart, blood vessels, urinary tract, kidneys, digestive tract, brain, and spine. These damages occur in up to 9 percent of babies born to mothers with type 1 diabetes and in up to 13 percent of babies born to mothers with type 2 diabetes. A woman may also have a stillbirth or spontaneous abortion, or a baby with major congeni-

Kimberly was diagnosed with type 1 diabetes eight years before she delivered her daughter and, two years later, her son—both beautiful, healthy children. Kimberly always wanted a family and knew she would do whatever it took to deliver healthy children, even when, while she was planning her family, the doctor gave her the news that she had diabetes.

"None of my doctors ever questioned my getting pregnant. They just said, 'Make sure you're in control beforehand.'" So, three months before she conceived, Kimberly started eating even healthier and became more rigorous about her exercise. While pregnant with the first baby, Kimberly switched from daily insulin injections to wearing an insulin pump. "Because sugars really fluctuate during pregnancy, the pump was the best way to have less peaks and better control. The first few months I needed a lot less insulin, and toward the end I needed three times as much.

"With my second child I set an alarm clock and checked my blood sugar every three hours. My doctors didn't ask me to do this, but I wanted to make sure I was doing everything to keep my blood sugar in good control. I also had so many ultrasounds and non-stress tests (NST) that my friends began to ask if something was wrong. It wasn't, and I wanted to keep it that way. I saw the extra tests as positive—I got to see my baby more often, probably a total of twenty-eight times from the thirtieth week on!"

tal malformations, macrosomia (larger than normal size), or respiratory distress.

Have an A1C test every one to two months before conception. Some physicians recommend that women switch from oral medications to insulin prior to and during their pregnancy for greater blood sugar control. A healthful diet and regular physical activity are just as important as ever if not even more important before, during, and after pregnancy. Some physicians recommend taking vitamin supplements and folic acid, a dietary supplement to decrease the chance of brain and spinal defects, one month before conceiving and during pregnancy.

Pregnant women with diabetes should see their doctor frequently and have frequent lab tests, because blood sugar during pregnancy is typically erratic. Some women will need to test their blood sugar at home as many as ten times a day, including during the middle of the night. Often a woman who is already using insulin will have to take extra insulin injections during her pregnancy. Insulin requirements toward end of term may be almost double, but at term, they usually drop again.

Gestational diabetes occurs during pregnancy

Gestational diabetes occurs in about 4 percent of pregnant women, typically between the twenty-second and twenty-eighth weeks of pregnancy. It is usually diagnosed during a routine screening for diabetes that women receive at the end of the second trimester. During pregnancy the placenta, an organ within the mother's uterus that attaches to the growing fetus and supplies nourishment, also produces hormones that at the end of the second trimester block the action of the mother's insulin. As the placenta grows, more of these hormones are produced and the insulin resistance increases, resulting in gestational diabetes.

Because gestational diabetes occurs after a fetus's body has already formed, the fetus is not prone to the same serious birth defects that occur early in pregnancy, those more commonly seen in babies whose mothers have diabetes before pregnancy. However, some women who are diagnosed with gestational diabetes actually had undiagnosed type 2 diabetes before getting pregnant. For that reason, it's important to have your blood sugar checked before conceiving. Women with gestational diabetes often deliver a large baby because the extra glucose in their blood travels through the placenta to the fetus, supplying it with more sugar than the fetus needs. The excess sugar gets stored as fat, resulting in a big baby. This extra weight can lead to breathing problems and future obesity or diabetes for your child.

Annie was diagnosed with gestational diabetes, but thinks she probably had type 2 diabetes before she got pregnant because her daughter was born with spina bifida, an open spine that forms within the first six to eight weeks of pregnancy as a consequence of high blood sugars. Also, after her pregnancy, Annie's blood sugars never went back to normal. More than 50 percent of Annie's family members on both sides, including eighty cousins, have diabetes. After Annie's daughter was born, doctors were able to close her spine, but Annie still wishes she'd had a blood sugar test before getting pregnant.

Treatment for gestational diabetes involves meal planning and physical activity, and some women will need to take insulin injections and test their blood sugars daily during pregnancy. Treating gestational diabetes helps lower the risk of a cesarean section at birth, which large babies often require. Gestational diabetes typically goes away after pregnancy; however, the American Diabetes Association recommends having your blood sugar levels checked six to twelve weeks after delivery to make sure they're normal. There's a 50 percent chance that if you've had gestational diabetes, you will go on to develop type 2 diabetes within five years. Maintaining a healthy weight and getting regular physical activity greatly reduce those odds.

MYTH #24

The stresses and strains of everyday life don't affect diabetes.

TRUTH: *Actually*, stress raises blood sugar, blood pressure, and blood fats and interferes with good diabetes management.

Stress is not healthy for anyone, but it has particular ramifications for people with diabetes. Whether physical (illness or injury) or mental (feeling under the gun at work, fretting over a sick child, etc.), stress increases your heart rate and raises your blood pressure, which can put you at greater risk for heart disease. It also stimulates appetite, interferes with sleep, causes sexual problems, and triggers anxiety, depression, and fatigue. All of this takes its toll on your body and your diabetes management. Chronic stress can even suppress your immunity and cause bone loss.

Perhaps the most surprising news, however, is that stress directly affects blood sugar. Richard S. Surwit, PhD, vice chairman of the Department of Psychiatry and Behavioral Sciences and chief of the Division of Medical Psychology at Duke University Medical Center in Durham, North Carolina, has studied the impact of stress on diabetes for more than twenty years. Surwit says that in people with diabetes, stress, depression, and general psychological state greatly influence blood sugar. The good news? Learning to control stress can actually have a positive effect on blood sugar.

How the fight-or-flight syndrome raises your blood sugar

Stress tricks your body into thinking it's under attack, so it goes into action preparing for combat or escape. This is commonly referred to as "fight or flight." In the days of our distant ancestors, when a hunter faced a saber-tooth tiger lurking in the woods, his body released stress hormones that induced an appropriate surge of energy to enable him to either fight the tiger or run away. Our bodies still respond in this same manner, only now it happens when we're stuck in traffic, worried about making a presentation at work, or even under chronic stress from going through a divorce. During a fight-or-flight scenario, blood pressure, heart rate, breathing rate, muscle tension, and blood flow to the muscles all increase. Stress hormones such as epinephrine (sometimes referred to as adrenaline) and cortisol are released to raise blood sugar in order to quickly boost the body's energy level, so sugar starts flooding the blood stream.

In people without diabetes, the pancreas recognizes this surge in blood sugar and responds by secreting more insulin, which shuttles the sugar into the cells, where it's used as energy. But when you have diabetes, you either lack insulin (as in type 1) or are not able to produce enough for your needs (as in type 2). Thus, during stressful situations, your blood sugar remains high. Stress hormones can also suppress the pancreas's ability to secrete insulin, further undermining your ability to blunt the rise in glucose.

Tip to Make You Tops

Whereas most people's glucose levels go up with stress, a small number of people's glucose levels actually go down. Why this happens is not well understood. Test your blood sugars when under stress so you can be sure what *your* body's reaction is.

Relaxation techniques can lower stress, and blood sugar

Imagine that you could protect yourself from going into fight-or-flight mode, that is from having a surge of stress hormones elevate your blood sugar. Dr. Surwit's quarter-century of research on the mind–body connection, along with numerous studies conducted by universities around the world, proposes exactly this. Just as our brain can set off the fight-or-flight response, it can also reverse the effect; the body's parasympathetic nervous system can slow heart rate, decrease blood pressure, and increase insulin secretion. "We now know," says Surwit, "that we can use the power of our mind to influence our body, including normalizing blood sugar levels."

In a Surwit study, 108 patients with type 2 diabetes learned a relaxation technique to help them cope with stress. After one year, those who continued the relaxation technique had a 0.5 percent improvement in their A1C (average blood glucose over the past two or three months). Although that seems a small improvement, Surwit says it's enough to reduce the risk for diabetes-related complications such as eye and kidney disease, and nearly a third of the people in the study experienced improvements in their A1C of 1 percent or more. Most compelling, says Surwit, the technique worked for everyone, including those who initially didn't report that stress was a major factor in their lives.

How to recognize when you're stressed

Unfortunately, stress has virtually become a way of life today, and many of us have grown so used to feeling anxious, with muscles tensed, that we're not even aware we're stressed. One way to notice that you're stressed is to log your blood sugars and see whether, when they are high, there's a stressful event going on in your life.

The American Diabetes Association suggests that before testing your blood sugar, you rate how stressed you feel by assigning a number between 1 and 10 to your stress level. Then test your blood sugar and write down your blood sugar level next to your mental stress number. After a week or two, look at your numbers and see whether you notice any pattern. Do you notice that when you wrote down a high stress level, you had a high glucose level? If so, it's safe to assume that at least some of your high blood sugars were stress-induced.

Remember, stress is not necessarily due to negative events. It can also be caused by something positive, such as excitement about your wedding, a trip you're looking forward to, or a job promotion. The first time I addressed a group of patients, I tested my blood sugar immediately afterward. I expected it to be low both before and after my talk because I hadn't had time to eat lunch beforehand. To my surprise, my blood sugar was 100 points higher than before my talk! When it happened a second time, I realized that my stress hormones had kicked in because of my nervous excitement and raised my blood sugar!

Tip to Make You Tops

To treat high blood sugar from stress: If you use insulin, take half the amount you would normally take to bring down your blood sugar. If you use oral medications, don't take more. These medications do not act quickly enough to compensate for the short-term effects of stress. Try taking a short walk instead.

Stress makes it harder to manage your diabetes

Short- and long-term stress and strain also take a toll on your diabetes management. Many diabetes care tasks tend to go by the wayside when you're stressed, and if you ignore your diabetes management, you put yourself at greater risk for developing diabetes complications. If one or more of the following phrases describe your recent behavior, try to take one small action to decrease and better manage your stress.

- Frequently forgetting to check your blood sugar levels
- Forgetting to schedule doctor appointments
- Not making time to shop for or plan healthful meals
- Eating on the run or reaching for unhealthful snacks
- Losing your appetite completely
- Drinking more alcohol than usual
- Cutting off social ties that provide support
- Feeling an overwhelming sense of pressure, loneliness, and a powerlessness to change things

Tips to reduce stress and minimize its effect on blood glucose

Dr. Surwit describes stress management as a fourth tool to manage diabetes (along with diet, exercise, and medication). Surwit recommends a therapeutic relaxation technique called progressive muscle relaxation (PMR) and writes about it in his book *The Mind–Body Diabetes Revolution*. PMR is a process of systematically tensing and relaxing the muscles in your body in a particular sequence. "A lot of us are walking around under a high level of arousal," says Surwit, "and progressive muscle relaxation helps people recognize when they're stressed and relax, which reduces their stress hormones and turns off their body's 'fight or flight' response." PMR creates an overall feeling of calm by deepening breathing, which can lower levels of stress hormones, blood pressure, heart rate, and blood sugar. The resulting reduction in blood glucose, says Surwit, can be just as effective as some medications for diabetes control.

Tip to Make You Tops

To practice progressive muscle relaxation (PMR), concentrate on one body part at a time. For instance, begin with your forehead, and tense the muscles there for about eight to ten seconds. Then relax those muscles and let all the tension go. Move progressively either up or down your body, tightening and releasing a muscle group. The more you practice, the more you train your parasympathetic nervous system to relax, so it will begin to do so automatically when you're in a tense situation.

My doctor manages my diabetes, so I don't have to concern myself.

TRUTH: *Actually*, although your doctor is responsible for your overall care, the daily management of your diabetes is up to you.

On a warm August day three years ago, I'd just finished delivering my first diabetes presentation in Easton, Pennsylvania, when a forty-something woman came up to me. "I got it!" she said excitedly. "When you said taking care of my diabetes is up to me, well, I never thought that before. I took my pills and then figured everything else was up to my doctor. But it is *my job* every day to do the things that will keep me healthy." She shook my hand vigorously and, smiling, walked out the door before I could even register how this simple concept would change her life—and her health.

With a short-term acute condition such as a sore throat or an ear ache, a health care provider diagnoses you, writes you a prescription, tells you to take your medicine, and two weeks later you're cured. That's hardly the case with diabetes. Diabetes is a chronic illness that must be managed on a daily basis so that it doesn't further endanger your health or impinge on your ability to enjoy life. Managing diabetes requires you to make everyday decisions about when, what, and how much you eat; getting physical activity into your day; taking your medicine; how to keep your blood sugar in target range even when you're sick or stressed; ensuring that you have enough supplies on hand; scheduling and keeping doctor appointments; and getting your lab tests done.

Tip to Make You Tops

Research shows that those who take charge of their diabetes, both physically and emotionally, do better overall than those who do not. When I give a presentation I tell the audience, "Your doctor doesn't sit down to dinner with you and whisper in your ear, 'Eat more broccoli and less French fries,' nor does he wake up with you and tell you to test your blood sugar—or if he does, I don't want to know about it!" It always gets a laugh, but more important, it gets the point across: *You* must manage your diabetes. You spend only a few hours a year with your health care providers; the other thousands of hours, your diabetes care is in your hands.

To learn more, take a diabetes class at a local hospital or get a referral to a diabetes educator or dietitian. Seek out books, magazines, Web sites, support groups, and health fairs for more information. The more you know, the more capable you will be to maintain good health.

You are an equal member of your health care team

At the 2008 annual American Association of Diabetes Educators conference, Dr. Bob Anderson, professor at the University of Michigan Medical School and a pioneer of the "empowerment approach," said that when it comes to diabetes, patients make 98 percent of the health care decisions. Further, diabetes educators are responsible not *for* patients but *to* patients, ensuring that patients can make informed decisions. Your health care providers are part of your wellness team, responsible for your overall care. They check

> ### *Tip to Make You Tops*
>
> Many people think they know when their blood sugar is high based on how they feel, but this generally isn't true. Testing your blood sugar is the only way to know whether it's in target range.

your vitals; provide information, guidance, and support; schedule tests; and offer strategies for improvement so that you can be successful managing your daily care.

You are also a vital member of this team. Your job is to evaluate the actions they recommend and determine how these actions fit into your life and goals. If it's comfortable for you to follow your health care provider's exact instructions, and if doing so gives you excellent results, then by all means do so. If, however, you prefer more freedom, flexibility, and control, and the best outcomes from your diabetes management, then it is in your best interest to learn all you can about diabetes.

Like so many other people, Saul believed that treating his diabetes was his doctor's job. "After all, I'm not a doctor. How could I possibly help?" he wondered. "I came from the generation where my parents believed that the doctors were always right.

"When I was diagnosed, all I was told was that in order to treat my diabetes, I should take my medication in the prescribed dose at the prescribed time—no questions, no exceptions." Medication alone and following such an unyielding plan didn't work well for Saul, so he took some diabetes classes and learned what would: regulating his physical exercise, eating healthy, carbohydrate counting, and stress reduction. Saul began practicing them all, and his A1C values have been in the 5's, the nondiabetic range, ever since.

Partnering with your provider on your treatment plan helps create success

In their book *The Little Diabetes Book You Need to Read,* nurse practitioner and certified diabetes educator Martha Funnell and former chairman of the American Diabetes Association Michael Weiss say that patients benefit when they help design their treatment plan and that a workable treatment plan meets the following criteria. It

- Takes into account your lifestyle, values, goals, resources, environment, and priorities
- Is workable for your life
- Is one you feel you can stick with
- Gives you a framework for the daily decisions that diabetes requires

The authors also recommend that following these four LIFE steps can help you, along with your health care providers, create a workable plan.

1. Learn all you can about diabetes and yourself.
2. Identify your three guiding principles: role, flexibility, and targets.
3. Formulate your self-management plan.
4. Experiment with and evaluate your plan.

It's easiest to make the types of life changes that diabetes may require if they are important to you and you believe you will be successful. Toward that end, build small steps into your plan so that you experience success. Each small success will lead to bigger steps and bigger successes. Also, commit to making a change gradually; for example, add physical activity to your routine a few days a week, rather than every day, at first. You'll find it easier to do.

LOOKING THROUGH THE LENS OF . . .
Betsy Rustad-Snell, Registered Nurse and Certified Diabetes Educator

Five Ways to Take Care of Your Diabetes

1. Be knowledgeable about your disease—get educated and stay educated! You can't manage diabetes unless you know how.
2. Trust your wisdom—once you've got the knowledge about diabetes, make wise decisions such as choosing healthful foods and getting daily activity. Not taking your insulin when you have type 1 diabetes is not being wise!
3. Find a mentor—someone who has well-controlled diabetes and a positive attitude. Once you have your diabetes under control, help someone else. Pay it forward.
4. Focus on the positive—as a result of having diabetes, you may end up eating better, getting more exercise, losing some weight, and having more energy.
5. Accept the fact that you have diabetes and seek support—from your family, your friends, and your faith. Remember, you are not alone.

Food Myths

There is one specific "diabetic diet" I should follow.

TRUTH: *Actually,* there is no longer any such thing as a "diabetic diet."

The same dietary guidelines recommended for all Americans are now recommended for people with diabetes: Eat a variety of vegetables, fruits, whole grains, lean protein, low-fat dairy, healthful fats, and fiber in appropriate portion sizes. No longer is there a recommended "diabetic diet," as there once was. You can even eat sweets; just make sure they are worked into your meal plan. An effective meal plan for anyone with diabetes is one that enables you

---

Tip to Make You Tops

Maudene Nelson, registered dietitian and diabetes educator at the Institute of Human Nutrition at Columbia University in New York City, calls the Plate Method for creating healthful meals "magic." Fill half your plate with any variety of colorful veggies low in carbohydrates, such as asparagus, broccoli, Brussels sprouts, eggplant, carrots, or cauliflower. Fill one-quarter of your plate with carbohydrate-dense foods such as potatoes, rice, beans, corn, or legumes, and fill the remaining quarter with lean protein such as chicken, fish, lamb, pork, or beef. Meals made with the Plate Method naturally contain a moderate amount of carbohydrates, little fat and cholesterol, and a good amount of fiber.

---

to keep your blood sugar, cholesterol, blood pressure, and weight within your target range, while allowing you to enjoy what you eat and not feel overly restricted.

Designing a healthful meal plan

A healthful meal plan should also address quantity, timing between meals, and the consistency of your carbohydrates—the food group that is primarily responsible for raising blood sugar.

Quantity—Most dieticians recommend that most women with type 2 diabetes get 45–60 grams of carbohydrate at each meal and most men 60–75 grams. The particular foods that you eat will probably vary, but to keep blood sugars level you should eat about the same *amount* of carbohydrate grams at each meal. For instance, if you eat cereal with milk for breakfast one day and a vegetable omelet the next, your blood sugars will be quite different as a consequence of the varying amount of carbohydrates in the two meals.

Timing between meals—A healthful meal plan offers choice regarding *when to eat*. Most people who eat regular meals spaced about four hours apart will not need to snack, because having regular meals helps keep blood sugars level. If you take medication that requires snacks, you may need to eat more often. If you use carbohydrate counting to match your medicine and carb intake, you will have maximum freedom regarding when you eat.

Consistency—A meal plan that works for you must be one you can stick with. Work healthful foods that you like into your carbohydrate allowance, and mix them up so you don't get bored. If you're craving something that's not on your meal plan but you just have to have it, have it and then go back to your plan. This helps keep you from binging.

Tip to Make You Tops

Through much of my twenties I tried to follow the "diabetic diet." To steer clear of a food I craved that wasn't on my meal plan, I'd reach for an allowable food such as a carrot, and then another such as half a grapefruit, and then a few more. Ultimately, I'd give in and eat whatever I was craving. You get the picture: lots of extra calories in the end. Today I go straight for a little ice cream or a cookie if that's what I want, recognize that it's allowed as long as I'm watching my blood sugar level and my caloric intake, and enjoy it.

Counting fat grams for weight loss and weight maintenance

Most people count calories to maintain or lose weight. Dietitian Megrette Fletcher advises counting fat grams instead: Eat the same number of fat grams for the *whole day* as you eat carbohydrate grams *at one meal*. Thus, if you're female and are allotted 45–60 carbohydrate grams at each meal, space 45–60 fat grams throughout your day. Stick to the lower end of that 45–60 gram range if you want to lose weight, and stick to the higher end to maintain your weight.

Tip to Make You Tops

To keep your carb and fat intake lower, stay away from "goo." Goo is any sauce that's gooey, whether in Chinese dishes such as this rule's namesake, Moo Goo Gai Pan, or cheese sauce, gravies, cream-based tomato sauces, and anything that comes out of the oven with a flaky, golden brown crust. "Goo" has at least fifteen grams of carb and lots of fat.

How fat, protein, and fiber affect blood sugar

Carbohydrates most alter blood sugar, but fat, protein, and fiber also play a role. Fat and protein have relatively little to no impact on raising blood sugar; however, they can slow down the absorption of carbohydrates. That's why many people find that when they eat pizza, for instance, their rise in blood sugar is delayed, and their highest blood sugar may occur four hours after their meal, not two. Having a "complex meal," one that combines fat, protein, carbohydrate, and fiber, helps stabilize blood sugar by slowing the release of glucose into the blood stream and promotes a feeling of fullness. It's pretty simple to create complex meals. A breakfast of Cheerios, milk, a peach, and sunflower seeds is a complex meal; it contains carbohydrates, protein, fat, and fiber.

Fiber also helps stabilize blood sugar. By slowing down the progression of food in the digestive tract, it blunts the release of glucose into the blood stream. Foods that have five or more grams of fiber per serving, such as beans, high-fiber cereal, lentils, pilaf, or bean spreads like hummus, help prevent rapid rises and radical drops in blood sugar.

Winning strategies to help you follow your meal plan

Even though the old restrictive diabetic diet has today morphed into a healthful eating plan, you may still need help at times *sticking* to your meal plan. Dietitian Fletcher recommends an eating strategy called "mindful eating." It helps break emotional eating habits. "Most people overeat to satisfy emotional hunger," says Fletcher. In addition, says Sasha Loring, a psychotherapist at Duke University Health System, "Most people don't think about what they're eating—they're focusing on the next bite." Both these habits make it hard to ever feel full. When you eat mindfully, you pay attention to what you're eating, consciously savor each bite, and learn to recognize whether your desire to eat is physical or emotional, which helps curb overeating and snacking.

In a randomized controlled trial at Duke and Indiana State University, binge eaters who participated in a nine-week mindful-eating program went from binging an average of four times a week to once a week and reduced their levels of insulin resistance. To practice mindful eating, slow down and really look at the food you're eating; notice its aroma, shape, color, texture, and taste. Enjoy the satisfaction of each single bite and tune in to how you feel while you're eating: Are you in a panic for more or calm and satisfied? For more information about mindful eating, go online to The Center for Mindful Eating's Web site at www.tcme.org.

Eating out is also a time when it's easy to go off your meal plan. You're not sure what ingredients or how much carbohydrate or fat are in a dish. Entrées are often larger than one portion size, and you may feel it's a time to throw caution to the wind and treat yourself. Here are a few of my strategies that allow me to have what I want and also stick to my meal plan.

- Make the server your ally—Ask (nicely, winningly, conspiratorially) if the restaurant can accommodate your dietary requirements.
- If the entrée comes with rice, pasta, or potatoes and you're watching your carbohydrates, ask whether they'll either double the green vegetable or substitute a salad for the carbs.
- Ask the waiter to "bring it on the side, please" for sauces, gravies, and salad dressings.

Megrette Fletcher, Registered Dietitian and Executive Director of The Center for Mindful Eating

Five Ways to Take Care of Your Diabetes

1. Try to eat meals that have three colors and three textures— foods that are colorful are high in vitamins and other nutrients. Also, eating foods that have a different look, feel, crunch, and taste makes meals more enjoyable.
2. Think about fueling your body much as you think of fueling a car, only in calories per hour. If you have a 200-calorie lunch, your tank will be empty in about two hours and you will be hungry again. Aim for eating enough calories to keep your body running efficiently: Don't run out of gas (calories) and don't overload.
3. Give yourself the gift of time. Take enough time to thoughtfully select, cook, taste, and enjoy what you are eating.
4. Notice your hunger before you eat. Take a minute before your next meal or snack, and ask yourself, "Am I hungry?" Considering this simple question can tell you whether your desire to eat is physical or triggered by something else.
5. Aim for consistency, not perfection. Make a consistent effort to eat well, rather than striving to have a "perfect" diet.

- Share an appetizer—My husband and I almost always do.
- Halve the entrée—If the portions are too large, ask whether they'll serve you half (and charge you half too!)
- Bag the dessert before it comes to the table. At a neighborhood restaurant where the prix fixe meal includes dessert, I

ask them to put it in a doggie bag straightaway so it doesn't come to the table to tempt me.

- Order what's not on the menu—Ask whether the chef will make you something you don't see on the menu with ingredients you do see.

Nine and a half times out of ten, my requests are honored with a smile. Restaurants want your business. If it's a neighborhood restaurant, let them know that if they accommodate you, they'll see you often.

MYTH #27

Healthful foods won't raise
my blood sugar.

TRUTH: *Actually,* foods that are healthful can also contain a lot of carbohydrates, which raise blood sugar.

Last year my friend Paula told me a humorous and poignant story about her neighbor who got type 2 diabetes a few months earlier. Paula's neighbor knew sweets such as cake, candy, and pie would raise his blood sugar, so he began asking his wife to fix a big bowl of fruit for him after dinner for dessert. He was shocked one night, when measuring his blood sugar after his fruit bowl, to discover that his blood sugar was over 300! Fruit is healthful, but it is also composed almost entirely of carbohydrates. Any food that contains carbohydrates, healthful or not, raises blood sugar and needs to be worked into your meal plan.

Carbohydrate, protein, and fat all affect blood sugar, but carbohydrate has far greater effect. Nor does it matter whether the carbohydrates come from "sweets" such as candy, cake, and pie, or from naturally sweet foods such as fruit, or from starches such as pasta, potatoes, and whole grains—your blood sugar level will rise based on the amount of carbohydrates in the food. Comparatively, protein has minimal effect on blood sugar. Only if you eat a great deal of protein will it have any noticeable impact on your blood

Tip to Make You Tops

When choosing fruits, remember that some raise blood sugar more than others. For instance, berries and melons, because they contain a lot of water, raise blood sugar less than bananas and mangoes. Dried fruits such as figs, apricots, and raisins contain approximately the same amount of carbohydrate as they do in their fresh state, but because of their smaller size you may be tempted to eat more of them, thereby consuming more carbohydrates (and calories).

sugar. Fat won't raise your blood sugar and, combined with carbohydrate, will actually slow its rise.

Healthful carbohydrates that raise your blood sugar

It may surprise you that ordinary nonstarchy vegetables such as broccoli and Brussels sprouts are half carbohydrate, but because their total amount of digestible carbohydrate is low, thanks to their high fiber content, they have a very small impact on blood sugar. Yet other healthful vegetables such as sweet potatoes, corn, beets, peas, and carrots contain a lot of carbohydrate. Dairy products such as yogurt, cottage cheese, and milk all contain carbohydrates and much higher amounts if you're choosing flavored yogurts or cottage cheese with fruit added.

Whole grains, which form the foundation of the USDA's food pyramid, are all carbohydrate, and beans, which are full of essential fiber, also contain significant amounts of carbohydrate. Even nuts and peanut butter (peanuts are actually a legume) contain carbohydrates, as do healthful whole wheat pastas and breads. The answer is not to avoid these foods, but to realize that they contain carbohydrate and to take that into account in your meal plan.

The exchange method and carbohydrate counting

To maintain blood sugar levels within your target range, even when eating healthful chunks of carbohydrate-rich pineapple, you need to match your medicine and the amount of carbohydrates you eat. One way to do this is by using the exchange method. Most common carbohydrate foods are assigned a number value based on their carbohydrate gram content and their effect on blood sugar. Foods of equivalent value are then "exchanged" for each other in your meal plan. For instance, one slice of bread, estimated at fifteen grams of carbohydrate, is considered one exchange. If your lunch meal plan calls for three carbohydrate servings, you can have two slices of bread and another food worth one carbohydrate exchange. Hmm . . . maybe two slices of that delicious pineapple.

Another method for matching your medicine and the amount of carbohydrates you eat is carbohydrate counting. This strategy is most often used by people who have type 1 diabetes. In this system, you first calculate the amount of carbohydrates in the food you will eat and then match your mealtime insulin dose to that amount of carbohydrates. This requires knowing how many carbohydrates are in the foods you typically eat and how many carbohydrates one unit of insulin covers *for you*. Some people with type 2 diabetes also use carbohydrate counting—this involves knowing how many carbohydrate grams you should eat at a meal, for instance forty-five grams, and what amount of the food you intend to eat equals forty-five grams of carbohydrate.

Tip to Make You Tops

The amount of insulin one needs to cover fifteen grams of carbohydrates is known as one's carb-to-insulin ratio and varies from
person to person. You can't go by what works for someone else. I
spent a weekend with two friends who both have diabetes, and by
eating the same foods and doing lots of blood sugar checks, we
discovered that each of us had a different carb-to-insulin ratio.

If you count carbohydrates, it's essential to know how to read
the Nutrition Facts label on packaged foods. Because all carbohydrates raise your blood sugar, you must use not the sugar content
but the total carbohydrate content, and make sure you're eating
one serving. Also, don't be fooled by foods labeled "sugar-free,"
"no sugar added," "reduced sugar," "dietetic," or "diabetic." Most
still contain carbohydrates, so check their label for total carbohydrate grams. If a food has five grams of fiber or more, however, you
can subtract the fiber grams from the total carbohydrate grams.
One word of caution: The U.S. Food and Drug Administration is
allowed a 20 percent margin of error when calculating carbohydrates, so if your meter results don't match a package's carbohydrate count, this may be the reason.

In addition to what you can learn from reading labels, many
books list the carbohydrate content of foods. I use *The Calorie King*.
The American Dietetic Association's Web site, www.eatright.org, offers nutrition information, and your health care provider may be able
to refer you to a dietitian or nutritionist if you need help working
with carbohydrates in your meal plan. You're best served if healthful
foods form the basis of your diet; just don't forget that those healthful foods have carbohydrates too.

I can't eat anything I like anymore!

TRUTH: *Actually,* you can eat anything, including your favorite foods.

I eat everything I love, including dark chocolate, chunky peanut butter cookies, and fried calamari, and so can you—unless a medical condition restricts you otherwise—by following two simple rules: (1) Eat smaller portions or indulge less often and (2) modify your favorite foods by substituting healthier ingredients for some of the sugars and fats. Thinking you can't eat anything you like anymore because you have diabetes is a mistake, yet diabetes educators and dietitians hear this lament all the time. If you want to eat something rich in carbohydrates or fat, you'll need to cut an equivalent amount of carbs or fat from somewhere else in your diet—you can eat *what* you want, just not *as much as* you want.

Megrette Fletcher, dietitian and diabetes educator, says patients can actually do themselves harm by assuming their food choices are limited. It's easy to begin to feel frustrated, angry, and disempowered, which then interferes with one's diabetes management. Fletcher tells her patients, "For many years you didn't have to pay attention to your diet and now you do, and that's hard, but it doesn't mean you can't eat what you enjoy or ever have a favorite food again. You can still have a serving of ice cream, just not all the time."

Tip to Make You Tops

If you're having food cravings, take a day or two off from your meal plan and cover a splurge with your medicine or exercise. The key is to strive to eat healthfully at least 80 percent of the time.

Familiarize yourself with portion sizes

Because portion control will enable you to eat whatever you want, become familiar with recommended portion sizes. One way is to read package labels. You may realize you've been eating far more than one portion serving. General guidelines, for instance, suggest two cookies, ten to fourteen potato chips, and a handful of M&M's as a serving size. Even when eating healthful foods, you should still follow recommended portions sizes: one-third or one-half cup for most grains and rice and one cup for green vegetables. Meats and poultry should be the size of a deck of playing cards.

Here are some "handy" guidelines for guesstimating portion sizes. After all, no matter where you go, you always have your hands with you.

- A woman's closed fist is about one cup of food; a man's is one and a half cups.
- Meat and protein should be the size of your palm.
- Sliced bread should be no thicker than your finger.
- A portion of cake should be about the thickness of your thickest finger. (In my house we call that a "sliver"—just enough of a taste to not feel deprived or guilty.)

- Round fruits such as apples, peaches, and plums are considered small if they can fit in your hand.

Reducing the amount of carbohydrates in foods

One alternative to eating less of your favorite foods is choosing their reduced-sugar versions. Here are some examples that can replace their higher-carb versions:

- Unsweetened apple sauce
- Artificially sweetened yogurt
- Low-sugar oatmeal
- Sugar-free ice cream
- Low-sugar jams and jellies
- Unsweetened canned fruit

Tip to Make You Tops

To save on carbohydrates, when putting out crackers and dip, replace half the crackers with thin slices of veggies such as squash, cucumbers, carrots, celery, and mushroom caps.

Reducing the amount of fats in foods

People with diabetes are at higher risk for cardiovascular disease, so it may be important to limit your fat intake. Choose lower-fat items, primarily monounsaturated and polyunsaturated fats rather than saturated fats and trans fats. Substitute lower-fat ingredients in recipes to help preserve heart health and avoid extra calories. Meals do not have to be high in fat to taste good. With a little creativity and experimentation, you can find substitutes for any favorite foods that are high in fat. Here are some ways to reduce fat, not flavor:

- Cook meat and poultry on a rack so the fat drains off.
- Use nonstick cookware or a nonstick spray instead of heavy oils or butter.
- Replace sour cream, mayonnaise, and margarine with their low-fat or nonfat versions. You can also substitute yogurt for sour cream.
- Steam vegetables and add herbs or light soy sauce rather than butter.
- Choose canola, corn, olive, sesame, almond, and peanut oil over hardened shortenings.
- Choose white skinless poultry over red meat.
- Rather than frying meat, poultry, and fish, bake, broil, roast, steam, grill, or braise them instead.
- Choose lower-fat cheeses such as feta, cottage, or Jarlsberg over higher-fat cheeses such as cheddar and brie.
- Replace ice cream with ice milk, low-fat frozen yogurt, sorbet, and Popsicles.
- Replace whole milk with low-fat or nonfat milk in cereal, puddings, soups, and baked goods, and for drinking.

Swap ingredients in recipes to lower carbohydrates and fats

The truth is that sometimes there's nothing that can replace a jelly donut or chicken fried steak, or so my friend in Texas tells me. During those times, give in and enjoy. But some ingredient swapping can allow you to still enjoy many of your favorite foods without noticing they're actually healthful. For instance, in many cake and muffin recipes you can cut the amount of sugar in half and add cinnamon, nutmeg, or vanilla to enhance sweetness. In baked goods that require moistness, bulk, and texture, replace the sugar with honey or molasses, and use less sweetener than called for. As a general rule, you can use less fat than recipes indicate and kick up the flavor with herbs and spices. For instance, Asian foods that typically have a lot of fat and salt can be made more healthful by using less of both and adding Asian spices such as scallion, ginger, and garlic. Of course, steamed chicken and broccoli is a perfectly healthful Asian dish. Here are some "old favorites" made new with more healthful ingredients:

Mashed Potatoes—Use half the amount of potatoes and an equal amount of turnips, rutabaga, or cauliflower. Add a little 2 percent milk, and top with a small amount of trans fat–free vegetable oil spread.

Sweet Potato Fries—Because white potatoes raise blood sugar even faster than table sugar, reach for sweet potatoes. Peel and slice lengthwise like steak fries. Toss gently with extra virgin olive oil and seasonings. Bake at 425 degrees for ten minutes on each side.

Crumb Coatings—Replace any flour or bread crumb coating with a mix of crushed nuts, seeds, and (unsweetened) whole grain cereal flakes. You can coat fish filets, chicken, shrimp, vegetables, or anything else you'd normally pair with bread crumbs.

Cold Cut Wrap—Roll sliced lunch meats or cheese inside a lettuce leaf rather than bread. Large, dark green or red lettuce

---

Looking Through the Lens of . . .
Susan Weiner, Registered Dietitian and Certified Diabetes Educator

Five Ways to Take Care of Your Diabetes

1. Use a "free food" to help make your meal plan more interesting. Foods such as salsa (for veggie dipping), sugar-free gelatin, or pickle relish provide very few carbohydrates and calories.
2. When dining out, contact the restaurant in advance. Many times the chef will be glad to speak with you and discuss the possibility of "kid-sized" portions or "low-carb" choices.
3. High blood pressure can often be controlled by reducing unnecessary sodium intake, so reduce your intake of processed foods, put the salt shaker back in the cupboard, and increase your use of spices!
4. Increasing dietary fiber helps stabilize blood sugar levels and lowers cholesterol. Opt more often for fiber-rich fruits and veggies and whole grain breads and cereals.
5. Foods with a lower glycemic index, such as beans, keep your blood sugar more level. Think about working with a registered dietitian to formulate a lower-glycemic meal plan.

---

leaves are also a great substitute for a burrito-size tortilla. If they aren't your cup of tea, use low-carb tortilla wraps.

Sautéed Mushrooms—Substitute these for half the breading in stuffing and half the ground beef in pasta sauce, chili, tacos, and burritos.

Ground Turkey—With less saturated fat and calories than lean ground beef, it works well in burgers, chili, meatloaf, tacos, burritos, Bolognese sauce, and meatballs.

Cauliflower Mac and Cheese—Substitute steamed, chopped cauliflower for half the macaroni in your favorite reduced-fat macaroni and cheese recipe.

Pita Pizza—Use whole grain pita, spread your favorite (sweetener-free) tomato sauce on it, add toppings and shredded mozzarella, and bake.

Soup—Try split pea soup or lentil soup for cold-weather comfort. They're thick and rich like corn soup and corn chowder with less glycemic impact.

It doesn't matter what I eat if I "cover" it with my medicine.

TRUTH: *Actually,* eating an excess of refined carbohydrates and un-healthful fats increases your risk of diabetic complications even if you do take extra medicine.

A friend with diabetes said to me recently, "I used to think the golden rule for managing diabetes was to eat anything and 'cover' it with in-sulin. A little extra insulin made birthday cake possible. A nutrition-ist showed me the error of my ways." It seems sensible to assume that if you want to indulge in sweets and fats, you can cover your excesses with extra medicine and do no harm. Most people in the medical community agree that you can—occasionally. But doing so with any frequency has two negative effects: (1) Taking extra medicine—certain diabetes pills and insulin—as well as consuming extra calories can lead to weight gain. (2) Weight gain tends to increase insulin resistance—the body's inability to use insulin efficiently. Most people with type 2 diabetes, and some with type 1, are already insulin resist-ant. Increased insulin resistance sets a vicious cycle in motion: Your blood sugar rises further, you need more medication to lower it, and this leads to more weight gain and more insulin resistance.

Further, weight gain and insulin resistance can cause elevated blood fats (HDL and LDL cholesterol and triglycerides) and high blood pressure. These four conditions together are known as metabolic syndrome. Metabolic syndrome puts you at greater risk for coronary heart disease, stroke, and peripheral vascular disease, which is a narrowing of blood vessels to the legs, arms, stomach, and kidneys.

Many people who take insulin follow the maxim my friend once invoked: *Eat a few more carbs, take a little more insulin.* After all, it's easy to put a few more units of insulin in your syringe or to program a little more insulin from your pump. But eating extra carbohydrates, particularly high-glycemic carbohydrates (carbs that increase blood glucose rapidly) has another effect; it tends to spike your blood sugar, causing another host of problems. Very high blood sugar is harder to control and bring down into target range, and you may overtreat your high blood sugar, making yourself susceptible to a low. When blood sugars swing up and down, you don't feel well physically, and you may also feel frustrated, angry, and depressed. Furthermore, many researchers and physicians think large swings in blood sugar are unhealthful and may increase the risk for diabetic complications.

The ADA's general dietary recommendation for carbohydrate is to eat no less than one hundred grams of carbohydrates daily; however, there is some controversy in the medical community about whether this amount is too high. For the first time in 2008, the ADA recognized that there may be some merit to lower-carbohydrate diets for those who want to lose weight.

Dr. Richard Bernstein, who has had type 1 diabetes for more than sixty years, is a noted advocate for a very low-carbohydrate diet. Bernstein believes many patients can achieve near "normal" blood sugars with an extremely low-carbohydrate diet. In his book *The Diabetes Solution,* Bernstein recommends that patients eat no more than thirty grams of carbohydrate daily. Eating twelve grams of carbohydrate at lunch and dinner and six grams at breakfast keeps weight down, requires less medication, and helps avoid blood sugar swings. Note that I didn't say it was easy!

Tip to Make You Tops

I follow a modified version of Dr. Bernstein's diet. I don't eat as few carbohydrates as he recommends, yet I removed the majority of refined carbohydrates from my diet after reading his book several years ago. Now that I've changed my diet, I take significantly less insulin, and my blood sugars are far easier to control. Major dietary change should be made under the care of your doctor or dietician.

Covering fats with medicine

Unlike with carbohydrates, you can't immediately "cover" the fat in a slice of triple brownie chocolate cake with a pill or injection. And although an occasional treat worked into your meal plan probably won't harm you, the frequent consumption of unhealthful fats will leave you more vulnerable to

- Weight gain
- Tissue inflammation caused by certain types of animal fat
- A need for cholesterol-lowering medication
- Heart and blood vessel disease that causes heart attacks and strokes
- Decrease in number of insulin receptors, increasing insulin resistance

Even though taking cholesterol medication helps guard against coronary heart disease, people with diabetes over the age of fifty are still four times more likely than people of that age without diabetes to have a heart attack and three times more likely to suffer a stroke. Recent research suggests that the age at which one is assumed to be at risk for heart disease should be lowered to forty-five. Teresa Hillier, MD, with the Center for Health Research at Kaiser Permanente, studied close to 8,000 eighteen- to forty-four-year-old men and women with type 2 diabetes and found not only that they suffered heart attacks and strokes at alarming rates, but also that, compared to adults who developed diabetes at a later age, they were 80 percent more likely to need insulin within two years of diagnosis.

Finally, consuming excess carbohydrates and fats can cause a condition known as "double diabetes." People with type 1 diabetes develop the problems commonly associated with type 2 diabetes, such as weight gain and insulin resistance, and people with type 2 diabetes exhaust their pancreas to the point where they no longer produce insulin. As one diabetes educator told me, occasionally indulging in a higher-carbohydrate or higher-fat treat or meal is probably fine, but the operative word is "occasionally."

When I feel the symptoms of low blood sugar, I should keep eating sweets until I feel better.

TRUTH: *Actually,* you should eat only fifteen grams of fast-acting carbohydrate and then check your blood sugar.

Years ago when I experienced hypoglycemia (low blood sugar), I would stand in front of my open refrigerator and proceed to eat everything in sight. My ravenous hunger and rapid heartbeat (two symptoms of hypoglycemia) and, to be honest, the excuse that now I *could* eat sweets, prompted me to devour anything sweet I could get my hands on: a handful of cookies, a piece or two of cake, a banana, raspberry preserves on toast . . . mmm. . . . I'd eat *all of this* while waiting for my blood sugar to rise. When I got a blood sugar meter some years later and started testing, I saw that my "eat-every-thing-sweet-in-sight" treatment gave me, an hour or so later, a blood sugar of about 350 mg/dl (19.4 mmol/l)! Today I know both from experience and from teaching others that the best way to treat low blood sugar is to (1) raise your blood sugar as quickly as possible and (2) do it in such a way that your blood sugar doesn't go above target range. That means following the Rule of 15.

The Rule of 15 is used as a guideline among diabetes health care providers; it's simple, is easy to follow, and will raise your blood sugar level quickly while keeping it within normal range. If you think you're experiencing hypoglycemia—symptoms include rapid heartbeat, weakness, headache, a cold sweat or clammy feeling, shakiness, irritability, dizziness, and hunger—check your blood sugar level. If your blood sugar is under 70 mg/dl (4 mmol/l), eat fifteen grams of fast-acting, simple, rapidly digested carbohydrate and wait fifteen minutes. Then recheck your blood glucose level. If your reading is still below 70 mg/dl (4 mmol/l), eat another fifteen grams of carbohydrate and test your blood sugar again in fifteen minutes. You want your blood sugar to be approximately 100 mg/dl (5.5 mmol/l).

If your blood sugar does not rise above 70 mg/dl (4 mmol/l) within thirty minutes after treating, get help. If a friend or family member is not nearby or easy to reach, call 911. Hypoglycemia should always be treated quickly to avoid an emergency situation, because an *extremely* low blood sugar level (below 30 mg/dl or 1.7 mmol/l) can cause loss of consciousness.

Each of the following items contains about fifteen grams of fast-acting, simple, rapidly digested carbohydrate.

- Four glucose tablets (available at a pharmacies)
- One tube of glucose gel, cake decorator gel, or glucose drink
- Half a glass of regular soda (not sugar-free)
- One to two tablespoons of honey or syrup
- Eight ounces of skim milk
- Six to eight Life Savers

If you're going to have a meal or snack within an hour, you don't have to do anything more. However, if your next meal is more than an hour away, have a snack of some carbohydrates with protein, such as a few crackers with cheese or peanut butter, to keep your blood sugar level up until your next meal.

It is very common to overtreat hypoglycemia as I used to do; low blood sugar causes stress hormones to be released that both stimulate hunger and make you feel jittery. To satisfy your appetite and calm the rising panic, most of us reach for food—too much of it and the wrong kinds. Candy bars, cake, cookies, pie, ice cream, and chocolate are a wholly ineffective way to treat low blood sugar, because the fat in these sweets slows down the digestion and absorption of the carbohydrates they contain. By the time your symptoms subside, your blood sugar will be far above normal range. "When patients tell me angrily that they're gaining weight and don't know why," said my friend Betsy, a diabetes educator, "I ask them if they're having a lot of lows. It's easy to forget all the calories you're eating if you're treating lows with cake and candy."

Tip to Make You Tops

If you're getting frequent low blood sugar readings, talk to your health care provider about changing your treatment plan. Learning how to count carbohydrates, eating a different amount of carbohydrates at meals, and snacking to better balance your medication may reduce the likelihood of hypoglycemia. Altering your medication and activity level may also help.

Hypoglycemia occurs when your blood sugar level drops too low to provide enough energy for your body's normal functioning. Typical causes include

1. Taking too much insulin or certain glucose-lowering oral medications (sulfonylureas, such as Glucotrol®, Amaryl®, Glyburide®, and Diabenese®; meglitinides such as Prandin® and Starlix®; or a combination drug such as Glucovante®, Avandamet®, or Metaglip®) for the amount of carbohydrates you have consumed.

2. A missed meal or snack.

3. Too much physical activity for the amount of carbohydrates and medicine in your system.

4. Drinking alcohol. (Refer to Myth #32: I shouldn't drink alcohol because it will raise my blood sugar.)

5. Variable absorption and action of insulin.

Ann, a diabetes peer-coach, was attending a diabetes conference when she ended up in the hospital with potentially life-threatening hypoglycemia. Just before stepping into the shower, Ann remembered it was time to inject her forty-six units of long-acting insulin. By mistake she took forty-six units of rapid-acting insulin instead! After living with type 2 diabetes for thirteen years, she simply made a very human error. "My dosing is so routine that I went through the motions without thinking," said Ann. Knowing the Rule of 15, and realizing that an overdose of forty-six units of rapid-acting insulin could have dire consequences, Ann yanked the fast-acting carbohydrates out of her hotel mini fridge, began drinking Coke, and checked her blood sugar every fifteen minutes.

Two friends took Ann to the hospital, where the attendants checked her blood sugar around the clock. Ann continued to consume carbs and was able to keep her blood sugar elevated. Within four hours she was holding steady at a blood sugar reading of 119.

6. Attempting to maintain tight blood glucose control. There's little cushion not to go below 70 mg/dl (4 mmol/l).
7. Human error, such as mixing up two different insulins.
8. Weight loss while on one of the oral medications mentioned in point 1. As you lose weight, your body becomes more sensitive to the insulin you're secreting.

Tip to Make You Tops

If your blood sugar has been high for some time and it begins to come down, you may experience what feels like (but probably isn't) hypoglycemia. My diabetes educator told me she always has a horrible day about a week after New Year's. "I start working out again and eating right, my blood sugar is dropping back into normal range, and I feel sick as a dog. I feel like I'm hypoglycemic, but my meter tells me I'm not. I know it's because my blood sugar is lower than where it's been for the last month enjoying all the holiday parties."

Using glucagon for treating dangerously low blood sugar

If your blood sugar goes so low that you lose consciousness, an injection of glucagon is the recommended treatment. Glucagon comes in a small kit you can purchase at the pharmacy; it stimulates the liver to release glucose into the blood stream and takes effect within five to twenty minutes. Most people with type 2 diabetes have a reserve of regulatory hormones that prevents their blood sugar from going excessively low, however, some conditions may put you at risk—having had diabetes a long time, having kidney or liver disease, or having frequent lows. If you have frequent low blood sugar episodes, speak to your health care provider about a prescription for glucagon.

People with diabetes should eat only sweets labeled "sugar-free" or "diabetic."

TRUTH: *Actually,* most of these foods are no better than ordinary sweets and may raise your blood sugar even more!

Many people believe that having diabetes means you can eat only sweet treats marked "diabetic" or "sugar-free," such as diabetic chocolate or sugar-free cookies. These items are marketed specifically to people with diabetes and are easily found on grocery store shelves and in gourmet sweet shops. However, according to the International Diabetes Federation, most diabetic foods in grocery stores offer no special benefits except perhaps to the huge food industry that reaps big profits from them.

Sugar-free and diabetic foods often contain just as many calories, carbohydrates, and fats as the sweets and other food products they replace. Furthermore, people with diabetes are not prohibited from eating sweets. What's important is to find a way to work sweets into a healthful meal plan so that they're a calculated part of your calorie and fat intake, and you still get most of your calories from healthful, nutritious foods.

Sugar-free and diabetic foods offer varying advantages

Besides the fact that sugar-free and diabetic food substitutes are generally more expensive, remember that a "sugar-free" food is not a "free food." A "sugar-free" food may not contain refined sugar, but it may contain as many calories and carbohydrates as the full-sugar sweet it's meant to replace, raising your blood glucose just the same. Beware: These sugar substitutes—corn sweetener, sucrose, high-fructose corn syrup, maltose, and fructose—contain carbohydrates. (Note: Any additive with the suffix "-ose" is a type of sugar.)

Tip to Make You Tops

Some sugar-free products contain sugar alcohol, a form of carbohydrate. Because these are not completely absorbed by the body, they have less impact on blood sugar and provide fewer calories. However, some can ferment in the intestines and cause uncomfortable bloating, gas, or diarrhea. If you have this reaction to a sugar-free product, check the list of ingredients. Malitol, xylitol, isomalt, sorbitol, lactitol, and mannitol are commonly used sugar alcohols.

You might not expect it, but sugar-free and diabetic foods may also contain a great deal of fat. Often, foods from which sweetening agents have been removed have fat added for a pleasing taste and texture. To get a real look at just how many calories, carbohydrates, and fat some popular sugar-free and diabetic foods contain, I went to my local grocery store and conducted my own market research study.

Note that you save only six calories by eating the sugar-free rather than the regular Oreos. The carbohydrate counts are the same, as are the fat counts. Comparing Murray sugar-free choco-

Comparative study of sugar-free and regular foods

	Sugar-free Oreos	Regular Oreos	Murray Sugar Free Chocolate Chip cookies	Chips Ahoy Chocolate Chip cookies
Price / Amount	$3.39/6.75 oz	$4.39/34 oz	$3.19/5.5 oz	$3.99/15.25 oz
Calories*	100	106	106	106
Carbohydrates*	16 g	16 g	13.2 g	14.6 g
Fat*	5g; 1.5 g saturated	5g; 1.5 g saturated	6g; 2.5g saturated	5.2g; 2g saturated
Sugar-substitute ingredients	Malitol, polydextrose, cornstarch, dextrose, sucralose, acesulfame potassium		Malitol, lactitol, polydextrose, sorbitol, sucralose	
Warnings on label	"Not a Reduced Calorie Food, Excess consumption may have a laxative effect"			

*Note: Amounts are based on a serving size of two cookies.

late chip cookies to Chips Ahoy, we see that Murray has slightly less carbohydrates and slightly more fat.

Tip to Make You Tops

Although sugar substitutes are not bad for you, nutritionist Megrette Fletcher says they don't taste particularly good, nor do they promote health. It's better to eat regular foods, such as fruit and real sweets, in moderation.

Kellogg's Special K is promoted as a healthful cereal that helps with weight loss, yet note below that, per serving, it has more calories than Kellogg's Corn Flakes and that, although it has less carbohydrates, it has more fat. It also costs more than a dollar more per box. Kellogg does, however, make a cereal called Special K Protein Plus that nets only 9 carb grams, 3 fat grams, and 100 calories per serving. Also, be sure to check a cereal's fiber grams: Corn Flakes gets a failing grade for fiber, whereas Cheerios receives high marks.

	Kellogg's Corn Flakes	Kellogg's Special K
Price / Amount	$3.39/12-oz box	$4.59/12-oz box
Calories*	100	120
Carbohydrates*	24 g	22 g
Fat*	0 g	0.5 g

Note: Amounts are based on a serving size of one cup dry cereal.

Smucker's sugar-free preserves, however, do appear to be a winner with less carbohydrates and less calories than regular preserves. Neither version contains fat.

	Smucker's Strawberry Preserves	Smucker's Sugar-Free Strawberry Preserves
Price / Amount	$2.49 / 12 oz	$4.59 / 12 oz
Calories*	50	10
Carbohydrates*	13 g	5 g
Fat*	0 g	0 g
Sugar-substitute ingredients		Polydextrose, maltodextrin, sucralose

Note: Amounts are based on a serving size of 1 tablespoon (17 grams).

Simple ways to cut down on sugar-free products

Consuming sugar-free products such as diet soda and artificial sweeteners in moderation is an easy and generally satisfying way to save calories. Here are a few simple and tasty natural substitutions:

- Add a slice of lemon or lime to carbonated or still water for zest.
- Use Stevia to sweeten hot and cold drinks; it's a noncaloric FDA-approved herbal sweetener available in health food stores.
- Try fruit and herbal teas because they have a slight sweetness and no calories.

Many sugar-free products offer few advantages when you are watching your weight and your intake of carbohydrates and fat. They're also typically more expensive. If you like these products or have a few special favorites, you can continue to use them, just read the label and choose wisely.

MYTH #32

I shouldn't drink alcohol because it will raise my blood sugar.

TRUTH: *Actually,* most alcohol works with your metabolism to *lower* your blood sugar.

Up until just a few years ago, there was scant information available about alcohol and diabetes, and since I'd been a bartender for a short time, I was, *ahem,* professionally curious. Any information I found said alcohol raises blood sugar. I was mystified, frankly, because I enjoy a glass or two of wine when out for dinner and I always find my blood sugar drops like a stone! Here's the real story: Most alcohol lowers your blood sugar. All alcohol begins as carbohydrates, such as potatoes, corn, or grapes. The fermentation process converts the sugar from the carbohydrates into alcohol, leaving little or no carbohydrates behind. Pure alcohol, whether gin, vodka, whiskey, scotch, or wine, does not raise your blood sugar; it typically lowers it, and that's because of how it's metabolized.

Normally when your blood sugar level starts to drop, your liver converts stored carbohydrate, called glycogen, into glucose. The liver then sends the glucose into your blood stream, which helps avoid or slow down a low-blood-sugar reaction. However, when alcohol enters your system, the liver's first job is to metabolize the alcohol so that it can be cleared from the body. While breaking down the alcohol, your liver is diverted from sending glucose into your blood stream. This process can take up to twelve hours or more, depending on how much you've had to drink. If you use insulin or an oral medication that prompts your pancreas to produce insulin, and possibly Byetta® or Symlin®, and you don't eat any carbohydrates while you're drinking, your blood sugar will probably drop and drop fairly rapidly. Eating carbohydrates while drinking is always advised to slow your blood sugar from dropping too fast and too far.

Tip to Make You Tops

Some research shows that a moderate amount of alcohol, when drunk with food, has little or no effect on glucose levels. A moderate amount is defined as one drink for women and two for men; one drink is defined as twelve ounces of beer, five ounces of wine, or one and a half ounces of hard liquor. However, you need to check your blood sugar to see how alcohol affects *you*.

Even those of us who've lived with diabetes for decades still have to pay extra attention so that our blood sugar doesn't go too low when we drink alcohol, and some of us have learned our lessons the hard way. My friend Miriam, who has type 1 diabetes and writes about diabetes for health publications, wrote about a pivotal night in her youth when she drank just shy of four beers. The next morning her roommate found her lying on the floor blathering incoherently—a sign of low blood sugar. Her roommate called 911, and when the paramedics tested Miriam's blood sugar it was below 20 mg/dl (1.1 mmol/l)! Because Miriam now lives alone with no roommate to intercede, she's learned to put certain safety measures in place. "I know I can't drink that much again," Miriam said, "and if I have a couple of drinks when I go out, I'll ask a friend to call me the next morning and make sure I'm okay. If I'm not at work by 10:30 A.M., I've also given my co-workers the green light to phone my apartment manager, who has keys to my apartment."

Tip to Make You Tops

Extend Bar, a nutritional snack created by pediatric endocrinologist Francine Kaufman, keeps blood sugar level overnight, when alcohol might otherwise lower it. The bar's primary ingredient, cornstarch, converts to glucose slowly and steadily over seven to nine hours. Extend Bars can be ordered online at www.extendbar.com or by phone at 1-800-887-2919.

The reason why many people think alcohol raises blood sugar is probably the effect of the mixer in a mixed drink. For instance, the Coke in rum and Coke, the orange juice in a screwdriver, and the sour mix in a Tom Collins raise blood sugar. Very sweet drinks such as dessert wine, liqueurs, and (for some people) beer will raise blood sugar. If you like a glass of wine with dinner, diabetes educator Kathy Spain says, "a moderate amount of alcohol may have heart-healthy and circulatory benefits, particularly in men over forty-five and women over fifty-five." However, she counsels patients against excessive drinking because it can cause liver disease, pancreatitis, some cancers, and hypoglycemia. Moreover, alcohol adds lots of unintended calories that you don't recognize while you're drinking.

Precautions when drinking alcohol

Drinking alcohol is a personal choice, but be smart about it. Here are several ways to protect yourself.

- *Snacking.* If you're not eating a meal with alcohol, have appropriate snacks. For instance, eat a few pretzels rather than nuts because pretzels have more carbohydrates, or mix a small amount of real soda or orange juice into a drink to help avoid low blood sugar. Be careful not to overdo it, however, or your blood sugar will go too high.

Tip to Make You Tops

When I have two glasses of wine with dinner, I make sure there's enough carbohydrate in my meal so my blood sugar doesn't drop too much, or I cut back on my insulin. I also check my blood sugar before going to sleep and make sure it's a tiny bit higher than usual to accommodate the drop in blood sugar that will occur overnight.

- *Hypoglycemia.* If you have a severe low-blood-sugar reaction that causes you to become unconscious, the normal remedy—an injection of glucagon—probably will not work if you've been drinking alcohol. Glucagon stimulates your liver to release extra glucose into your blood stream, but alcohol blocks this process. Do your best to avoid this scenario by testing your blood sugar frequently, taking precautions against low blood sugar, and ingesting glucose tablets or gel if your blood sugar is dropping.

The best way to avoid extreme highs or lows is by testing your blood sugar shortly after you finish drinking, again several hours later, before bed, and when you wake up, because alcohol can lower your blood sugar through the night and into the next morning. If you've had a lot to drink and you take a basal (long-acting) insulin before bed, you might lower your dose.

- *Wear a medic alert bracelet.* The symptoms of hypoglycemia—shakiness, muddled thoughts, irritability—can make it appear that you're drunk. If you experience hypoglycemia, you want someone to treat you for low blood sugar, not for being drunk.

- *Never drink and drive.* Not only will you not have your full faculties behind the wheel, but you could have a hypoglycemic event and kill yourself or someone else.

- *Complications.* Alcohol can worsen some diabetic complications, such as eye disease and high blood pressure. It can also raise triglyceride levels and is particularly toxic to nerves, which can make burning, tingling, and numbness of peripheral neuropathy worse.

- *Medicine.* Be careful about the effects of combining alcohol with any medication you are taking. Ask your health care provider specifically about the medicine you take and its interaction with alcohol. Metformin (brand name Glucophage®), specifically, should not be taken by anyone who drinks excessively. Mixing alcohol and metformin can lead to a severe and dangerous metabolic reaction.

- *Weight gain.* Alcohol can significantly add to weight gain. A drink averages around one hundred calories (more for mixed drinks), and drinking tends to increase your appetite while lowering your resolve to stick to your meal plan.

Body Fitness Myths

MYTH #33

I have to lose a lot of weight for my diabetes to improve.

TRUTH: *Actually*, a modest weight loss can improve your blood sugar, blood pressure, and blood fat levels and can reduce your risk of diabetic complications.

You may have heard it from your doctor a million times: "Lose weight and get more exercise." And you may have tried to do it just as many times, or so it feels. What is seldom told to patients, however, is that although getting your weight to a healthy range is ideal, numerous benefits are achieved just by losing 5 to 10 percent of your body weight. In other words, you don't have to lose a *lot* of weight to improve your blood sugar control and lower your blood pressure, cholesterol, triglycerides, need for medication, and risk of diabetic complications. Losing just ten to fifteen pounds, studies show, creates these improvements for many people, in addition to lightening the load on your hips, knees, ankles, and feet, allowing you to move around and breathe more easily, and giving you more energy.

While there are contrary opinions as to whether excess weight causes insulin resistance or insulin resistance causes excess weight, most people who get type 2 diabetes are overweight and losing weight is usually the first step recommended for managing type 2 diabetes.

The study "Meta-analysis: Effect of Dietary Counseling for Weight Loss," published in the July 2007 issue of *Annals of Internal Medicine,* shows that losing about 5 to 7 percent of one's body weight can decrease insulin resistance, help normalize blood sugars, and reduce the risk of short- and long-term complications by as much as 40 percent. The American Diabetes Association's standards of care recommend losing this much weight as a starting point to improving glycemic control. Those who are obese may need to lose more weight to reap these benefits, but accomplishing this smaller weight loss, diabetes educators say, helps inspire patients to go on and make larger improvements.

Measures of weight and fat to improve your health

The first simple measure on your way to regaining health is to check your weight against a standard weight chart, comparing your actual weight to the ideal weight for your height and frame. The average 5 foot 4 inch American female should weigh about one hundred and thirty-three pounds, with a range between 114 and 152 pounds. The average 5 foot 8 inch American male should weigh about one hundred and fifty-four pounds, with a range between 137 and 171 pounds. Many Web sites, such as www.healthchecksystems.com/heightweightchart.htm, have a reference chart. Your body mass index (BMI) is also an important number to know. It tells you what percent of your body weight consists of fat and is calculated according to your height and weight. A normal BMI falls between 18.5 and 24.9. A BMI between

25 and 29.9 is considered overweight, and one above 30 obese. Again, the best way to calculate your BMI is using an online calculator, such as the one found at www.nhibisupport.com/bmi/.

Although total body fat is important, most obesity experts consider *where* fat tissue is located on your body to be the main predictor of weight-related diseases such as atherosclerosis and heart disease. Abdominal fat is the most dangerous. If you are apple-shaped, meaning you carry most of your weight around your stomach and abdomen, you have a greater risk of weight-related disorders than if you are pear-shaped and carry more of your weight on your buttocks and thighs. People with an apple shape are thought to have a higher risk of elevated blood pressure, triglycerides, and LDL (bad) cholesterol; low HDL (good) cholesterol; heart disease; and stroke. Waist circumference can help determine whether you are an apple or pear shape. Measure your waist just above your belly button. If you are male, a healthy waist measurement is less than forty inches. If you are female, a healthy waist measurement is less than thirty-five inches.

Aging and hormones can often cause fat buildup around the abdomen, but losing weight may affect your shape, as may tar-

---

Tip to Make You Tops

The importance of exercise and physical activity cannot be overstated both for weight loss and for loss of abdominal fat. In studies on identical twins who have a tendency to be overweight, scientists found that physical activity was the strongest determinant of total body fat and central abdominal fat.

geted exercises. Want to shake some of that belly fat away? No kidding: Try belly-dancing!

How to lose 5 to 7 percent of your body weight and keep it off

Going on a crash diet, eliminating every fat or carbohydrate from your diet, eating only green, purple or red foods, or eating upside down is *not* the way to lose weight healthfully or to maintain weight loss. You're almost guaranteed to put back whatever weight you lose, and more, when you go off your restrictive regimen. Reaching a healthy weight safely and maintaining it for the rest of your life call for healthful lifestyle habits and for setting a modest, achievable goal of losing one or two pounds a week.

I'm not saying by any means that it's simple to lose weight. I am saying you can accomplish it simply if you follow these guidelines: (1) Improve your diet to include more nutritious foods, (2) eat single servings of a food, and (3) increase your physical activity. In addition, a successful weight loss plan should be

1. Workable whether you're at home, at work, or traveling
2. Maintainable for the rest of your life
3. One that keeps your blood sugars within target range most of the time, including two hours post-meal blood sugars

If you need help devising a meal plan, ask your health care provider for a referral to a dietitian or nutritionist. An exercise physiologist can help you safely get more activity into your day.

Here are some helpful steps to weight loss:

- Make your goal realistic—Plan to only lose five, ten, or fifteen pounds over a reasonable amount of time. Don't think any further.
- Keep a food diary—Write down what you eat. According to one of the largest and longest-running weight loss trials ever conducted (by Kaiser Permanente's Center for Health Research), writing down what you eat, identifying your habits, and making small changes can double your weight loss.
- Create a health-friendly house—Clear the junk food out of the cupboards and stock up on fruits, vegetables, and whole grains. It's a lot easier to eat the right things when they're readily available in place of unhealthful foods.
- Eat nutrient-dense foods—These are foods rich in nutrients and low in calories, such as green vegetables, whole grains, beans, and fruits. You'll get more nourishment and fewer calories and, over time, lose your craving for high-fat, high-sugar foods.
- After-dinner treats—Decide that any snacking after dinner will be on only healthful foods.

Tip to Make You Tops

"The Daily Plate" section of the Web site www.livestrong.com provides information, support, and food and fitness tools to accomplish your weight goals. You'll find calorie counts, read about your habits and patterns, and access a cheering support group.

- Add one physical activity to your day each week—Climb the stairs at work, park farther away, or walk after dinner.
- Pick a workout that works for you—If walking is hard for you, try exercising in a pool or lifting weights.
- Check your medications—If your diabetes medications cause weight gain, find out whether you could benefit from medications that actually help most people lose weight, such as Byetta® and Symlin®, or Januvia®, which is weight neutral.
- Follow the 80/20 rule—If you "eat healthy" and get moderate activity 80 percent of the time, you're doing great!

Exercise isn't important for managing my diabetes if I'm taking medicine.

TRUTH: *Actually*, even if you take medication, physical activity helps you better control blood sugar, aids in weight loss, and makes insulin more effective.

Physical activity is especially important for people with diabetes, regardless of whether they take medication. In fact, regular physical activity, a healthful diet, and medication form the cornerstones of managing diabetes. Numerous research studies show that people with type 2 diabetes who exercise tend to have blood glucose levels in their target range more often and are able to lose weight and keep it off more easily than those who don't exercise. These two all-important aspects of managing diabetes can help increase the odds of delaying or preventing such diabetic complications as heart attack and stroke, foot and lower-extremity problems, and eye and kidney disease. People with pre-diabetes also reap the same benefits from regular physical activity. In addition, regular physical activity

- Decreases "bad" (LDL) cholesterol and increases "good" (HDL) cholesterol. Both are risk factors for heart disease, and two out of three people with diabetes die from heart disease and stroke.

- Reduces high blood pressure, which afflicts nearly half of all people with type 2 diabetes.
- Increases blood circulation for bone and tissue health, particularly in your feet where circulation can be poor.
- Builds muscle, and muscle burns more calories than fat, even at rest!
- Gives you more energy throughout the day.
- Improves the quality of your sleep and helps you manage stress.

Exercise is so beneficial to good diabetes management that Lois Exelbert, registered nurse and administrative director of the Diabetes Center at Baptist Hospital in Miami, Florida, says patients who diligently monitor their blood sugar, watch their diet, and take their medicine, yet don't exercise, won't get the same benefits from their treatment. "Without exercise, the other things on the list really don't work very well," Exelbert says.

Tip to Make You Tops

Exercise aids weight loss, and many people who get regular physical activity and lose weight are able to reduce their medication or, in some cases, eliminate medication altogether.

I have talked with many people with diabetes who have added a moderate amount of physical activity to their day and have seen improvements in their blood sugar, blood pressure, cholesterol, weight, and outlook on life. Philip was seventy-three when he got diabetes. His doctor put him on Avandia®, which helped bring down his blood sugar from 400 mg/dl (22 mmol/l) to 200 mg/dl (11 mmol/l), but Philip wanted to control his blood sugar with diet and exercise alone. "I started watching what I was eating, and my wife and I began taking a thirty- to forty-five-minute walk most evenings after dinner," he explained. Now Philip is controlling his blood sugar without medication and, whenever he doesn't take his walk, notes that his blood sugar is higher than usual the next morning.

Mel, a fifty-nine-year-old photographer, finds that his blood sugars have been better controlled since he began using the stairs at work instead of the elevator. Ann, a retired schoolteacher, has worked up from ten-minute to forty-five-minute evening walks with her husband. They go three or four nights a week after dinner, and her A1C level has come down from 8 percent to under 7 percent. Greg, who got diabetes eight years ago at age thirty-seven, was overweight and headed for a heart attack. He began hiking with his daughter near his Virginia home, shed pounds, and lowered his A1C several points to 5.7 percent! Now every Sunday is reserved for a loving father-daughter hike.

Tip to Make You Tops

When I hurt my ankle in 2008 and couldn't take my power-walk for three months, I saw how much exercise does for me. I had to increase both my Lantus® (long-acting insulin) and my Humalog® (rapid-acting insulin) several units, even, while my diet stayed exactly the same. And I gained four pounds—crystal clear evidence that regular exercise can help reduce your medication and control your weight.

Two of my fellow diabetes peer-coaches, Stephan and Saul, were both one hundred pounds overweight when they were diagnosed with type 2 diabetes at ages forty-one and fifty-one, respectively. Neither was a fitness enthusiast, yet both began exercising as a way to manage their diabetes. Stephan was a retired army sergeant but he'd grown slow and sluggish, and at diagnosis his A1C was a whopping 16 percent! Today he has participated in several triathlons, his A1C is 6.5 percent, and he's regained his former confidence. Stephan says exercise and frequent testing make the biggest differences to his management.

Tip to Make You Tops

Most people need information, motivation, and support when beginning an exercise program. The Diabetes Exercise and Sports Association (DESA) is an organization dedicated to teaching healthful and safe exercise strategies for the treatment of type 1 and type 2 diabetes, and for the prevention of type 2 diabetes. DESA holds an annual conference every spring where exercise professionals, athletes, and people with diabetes come together to share knowledge and enhance their physical fitness.

Fit4D, at www.Fit4D.com, is an online service that provides guidance, coaching, and support from diabetes educators, nurses, exercise physiologists, dietitians, and personal trainers. They can help you design, and stay on, a fitness program or reach new goals.

Saul, fearing complications upon diagnosis fifteen years ago, vowed to get his blood sugar in the nondiabetic range (an A1C of between 4 and 6 percent). Saul began riding a bicycle and today, at age sixty-nine, rides ninety miles a week, has significantly reduced his medication, has no complications, and has an A1C of 5.3 percent. Saul rides with three bike clubs, one of which is a mentoring program for teenagers, and he says his bike buddies keep him going with their endless support.

Even though some people transform themselves from couch potatoes into athletes, it's not necessary for reaping many of the advantages of exercise. Just incorporate more activity into your day with greater regularity: Climb a flight or two of stairs, walk five blocks for a quart of milk instead of taking the car, spend twenty minutes walking the dog rather than ten, and throw yourself into cleaning the house, knowing how beneficial the physical activity is for your heart, your weight, and your blood sugar. Gary Scheiner, an exercise physiologist (a professional specifically trained in how exercise interacts with the body's structure and function) says not only does fitness improve our diabetes health, but that any activity that improves overall fitness—even if it is undertaken in small steps—also motivates people to take better care of themselves and their diabetes.

An exercise prescription from the experts

How Often to Exercise: Experts recommend physical activity for thirty minutes a day at least five days a week, and here's why: When a muscle is exercised, it draws sugar out of the blood stream for fuel, which helps control the level of sugar in the blood. This effect can continue for between twelve and (as much as) seventy-two hours afterward, depending on how vigorously and how long you exercise. By exercising every day or every other day, you make this regulation of glucose continuous.

How Long to Exercise: If you're new to exercise, start slow; doing too much too soon often leads to injuries and defeat. Delaine Wright, clinical exercise physiologist and diabetes educator, says that unless you have an orthopedic limitation, you should start with simple walking five or ten minutes at a time, three times a day. Within a few weeks, do a continuous twenty- to thirty-minute walk. If using a bicycle, do ten or fifteen minutes at the start. If using weights, begin with ten repetitions and slowly increase over several weeks. Over time, extending any of these activities to forty-five or sixty minutes can be more beneficial, particularly for weight loss.

What Constitutes Exercise: Any physical activity that engages your large muscles, elevates your heart rate, and increases your

---

Tip to Make You Tops

Physiologist Delaine Wright advises that you learn your body's response to exercise through frequent testing of your blood sugars, including before and after an exercise session or activity. If you walk thirty minutes a few times a week, test within the first ten minutes after ending your walk one day, half an hour after your walk another day, and one hour after your walk a third day. The following week, do the same, using two-, three-, and four-hour interval checks. Look at your blood sugar numbers as the result of an experiment, says Wright. "You won't be disappointed when you see, after a half-hour walk, that your blood sugar came down fifty points!" If you use insulin or glucose-lowering medication, there may be certain adjustments you'll have to make with your medicine or diet to best manage your blood sugar. (For further information, refer to Myth #37: It's not safe for people with diabetes to exercise or play sports.)

breathing is beneficial. This includes aerobic exercise, weight train-ing, and many activities you already do, such as vacuuming and raking the leaves.

Tip to Make You Tops

Check the Centers for Disease Control and Prevention (CDC) Web site, www.cdc.gov, for a breakdown of light, moderate, and vigorous activities.

Here's a list of recommended activities:

- Walking
- Swimming
- Biking
- Jogging
- Cleaning the house
- Taking a group exercise class
- Rowing
- Cross-country skiing
- Ice skating
- Jumping rope
- Dancing
- Hiking
- Mowing the lawn
- Taking the dog for a long walk
- Climbing stairs
- Pushing a stroller
- Walking nine holes on a golf course

Delaine Wright, Registered Clinical Exercise Physiologist and Certified Diabetes Educator

Five Ways to Take Care of Your Diabetes

1. Use your blood glucose meter as a motivational tool by checking before and after exercise—you will be amazed at the power of exercise to lower your numbers. Knowing that your blood sugar can come down significantly after a half-hour walk helps push you out the door to do it.
2. Pick one day every two months to try a different activity. Sign up for a ballroom dance class, go for a group hike, bird watch, or learn how to kayak.
3. If on an insulin pump, pattern your blood sugar response to exercise by mimicking what the nondiabetic pancreas does during exercise. You may have better results by reducing your basal a half-hour before moderate activity and resuming normal basal levels 20 minutes prior to stopping.
4. There are many options and approaches to taking care of your diabetes through nutrition, exercise, and medications. Work with your health care team to find the best options *for you.*
5. Make diabetes fit your life, not the other way around, and know that diabetes can *better* your life, inasmuch as it encourages eating more healthfully and appreciating what you have.

How to Exercise with a Physical Limitation: If you have any limitation from a coexisting medical problem, ask your doctor to suggest an exercise you can do. Also, having a diabetes complication such as neuropathy does not mean you can't be physically active. It may just mean you have to make modifications to equipment or adaptations in certain activities. Some recommended activities are swimming, bicycling, rowing, chair exercises, arm exercises, yoga, and t'ai chi. An exercise physiologist can also help you identify an activity you can manage and instruct you in protecting your joints and skeletal structure.

How to Exercise If You Hate Exercise: Maybe you haven't done any physical activity in so long it seems overwhelming, or your extra weight makes even a short walk tiring. Maybe you have terrible memories of being the last one picked in high school for the volleyball team (don't ask!). But just start moving a little more, and you'll feel better *and* feel you have more control over your diabetes. Pick something you enjoy so you'll stick with it, and if you get bored, mix it up: Walk two days a week, ride a bike one day a week, and spend Saturdays working in the yard.

MYTH #35

If anything were really wrong with my foot, it would hurt.

TRUTH: *Actually,* because diabetes can cause you to lose sensation in your feet, you may have a foot injury and not know it.

One of the most common complications of diabetes is peripheral neuropathy, which causes pain or loss of sensation in your hands and feet. When you have peripheral neuropathy—which usually begins in the longest nerves, such as the ones that reach to your toes— sensory information relayed from your nerves to your brain doesn't get transmitted. This means that thoughts such as "My feet are cold" and "Ouch—I burned my finger" don't actually register in your brain. Such a loss of feeling in your feet makes them less sensitive to pain, heat, and cold, and you may experience numbness, tingling, burning, or stabbing sensations. Thus, you *can* have a foot injury and not know it.

Birgitta Rice, a foot care specialist, told me a pretty amazing story: "I once saw a patient who had walked around all day with a model toy in his shoe and had no idea. He told me that when he put his shoe on that morning it felt a little odd, so he adjusted his sock. That night when he took his shoe off, the toy fell out. He hadn't felt it at all!" Many people walk barefoot on hot sand and burn their feet. Still others have walked around with a staple, tack, or nail that has gone right through their shoe and their *foot,* without knowing it's there.

Kathleen shared with me her story of unknowingly stepping on a staple eight years ago, an injury that led her to a wound clinic and, months later, necessitated the amputation of her big toe. "It was nine o'clock at night and the doorbell rang. I got up from the sofa and walked across the living room floor to answer the door. It was a pizza delivery—and it was for my upstairs neighbor!" Kathleen had no idea she'd stepped on a staple during her walk to answer the door until that night when she took off her sock and saw the blood.

Foot problems can lead to amputation

If you lose sensation in your feet, you can easily develop a foot ulcer, and the more you learn about foot ulcers, the more you want to make sure you never get one. A foot ulcer is a breakdown of the top layer of your skin and is the foot injury that most commonly leads to amputation. A foot ulcer first appears as an open sore on your foot, and, if it is not treated, an infection can make its way into the tissue of your foot and then the bone. If you've lost feeling in your foot, you can walk around with a deep ulcer and not know it. The most common risk factors for ulcers are diabetic neuropathy and structural foot deformities. The good news is that, as in most things involved in diabetes, an ounce of prevention is worth a pound of cure: If you're at risk for foot ulcers, practice good foot hygiene, including proper nail care and wearing protective footwear to reduce the risk of injury, which can lead to a foot ulcer. If you detect a foot ulcer early, you can usually heal it with antibiotic cream, but foot specialist Rice advises that you check with your doctor before doing anything on your own.

Even a blister from wearing a shoe that you can't feel is too tight, if left untreated, can lead to an infection. Blisters can easily turn into foot ulcers. Podiatrist Dr. Joseph Stuto points out that having diabetes puts you at risk for foot problems due to poor circulation, and your autoimmune system may also be compromised to fight infection. "It doesn't mean you're going to have a problem," says Stuto, "but the better you keep your blood sugar, cholesterol, and blood pressure, the better you're going to do."

Tip to Make You Tops

An exceptional video called *If You Have Diabetes™*, produced by Alpyn Health Education, provides information and moving testimonials about living with diabetes and diabetic foot problems. You can order a copy by going online to www.alpyn.com.

A loss of sensation can cause foot deformity

If your feet lose feeling, they are also at risk for deformity. This can come from an infected foot ulcer or open sore, a change in the arch of your foot from the normal pressure of everyday walking, neuropathy, or muscle loss that contributes to the breakdown of bones in your foot, causing a bone condition called Charcot (pronounced "sharko") foot. This is one of the most serious foot problems associated with diabetes, wherein the foot becomes misaligned and deformed as a consequence of a lack of nerve stimulation, and muscles that can no longer support the foot properly. The result is that bones fracture and disintegrate. Charcot foot is so severe that it can change the entire shape of your foot, but because your foot doesn't hurt, you may continue to walk on it, worsening the condition.

Tip to Make You Tops

To ward off foot ailments, it's vital to keep the muscles in your feet and legs strong. Simple walking, says foot specialist Birgitta Rice, is one of the easiest and most effective ways to do this.

How to do a foot inspection

The ultimate consequence of an undetected, untreated foot problem can be the amputation of a toe, foot, or leg below the knee. If you can't feel your feet, look at them every day to check for blisters, bunions, cuts, or anything unusual, and seek help right away if there are abnormalities. If you've lost feeling in your feet use your eyes and hands to help you detect a problem. You should also inspect the tip of your big toe, the base of the little toes, between your toes, your heel, the outside edge of your foot, and across the ball of your foot every day. Look for puncture wounds, bruises, pressure areas, redness, warmth, blisters, ulcers, scratches, and nail problems. Feel both of your feet for possible swelling. If you can't see your feet, use a mirror or have someone help you. The importance of inspecting your feet can't be overstated: Even little things like cutting your toe nails improperly because you can't reach them can create unnecessary problems.

See your doctor or podiatrist on a regular basis, at least annually and more often if necessary. Take your shoes and socks off when you're sitting on the examining table in your doctor's office to remind him or her to examine your feet. Keeping your eyes on your feet is the surest way to see that they stay where they belong—right there at the end of your body.

Tip to Make You Tops

Foot complications don't usually occur in children with diabetes. However, because it can be hard for a child to communicate a problem with his or her feet, establish a routine of inspecting your child's feet regularly. Make a game of it so it's fun rather than frightening: "*This Little Piggy*," for instance, is an ideal way to make a foot inspection fun. As children get older, pass foot inspections on to them, but still keep an eye out for any changes you might notice in their walk, activity level, or posture.

My vision is blurry because I'm getting older.

TRUTH: *Actually,* that's possible, but blurry vision can also be a sign of high blood sugar or diabetic eye disease that, if left untreated, can lead to vision loss or blindness.

When Sally noticed that her vision was blurred, she went to her general practitioner expecting he'd send her to the eye doctor to be fitted for glasses. After all, her brothers and sisters all wore glasses; naturally, she would too. Because Sally was overweight, her physician asked her whether she'd ever had her blood sugar checked. She had, but that was long ago when she'd had gestational diabetes during her pregnancy. Her doctor did a blood sugar check in his office, and Sally's blood sugar was 435! A month of diet, exercise, and diabetes medication brought Sally's blood sugar back under control and her vision back to normal. Blurry vision is one of the most common symptoms of high blood sugar.

Blurry vision can also be a symptom of a diabetic eye disease, a complication of diabetes. Because high blood sugars can weaken the small blood vessels behind the eye, diabetes puts you at greater risk for eye diseases that can cause vision loss and blindness. The most common of these are glaucoma, fluid pressure inside the eye that leads to optic nerve damage and vision loss; cataracts, clouding of the eye's lens; and diabetic retinopathy, damage to the blood vessels that supply oxygen to the retina.

What you should know about glaucoma

Glaucoma is a condition caused by a reduced level of oxygen reaching the eye, which forces the eye to form new blood vessels. These new blood vessels may cause scarring and block normal drainage of the eye, which then causes pressure to build up in the eye. The Nurses' Health Study, a twenty-year study of 76,312 women, found that women with type 2 diabetes have approximately a 70 percent increased risk for the most common form of glaucoma, called primary open-angle glaucoma. Neovascular glaucoma, a more rare glaucoma, has also been directly linked to diabetes. Depending on the type of glaucoma, treatment may include medication, prescription eye drops, or surgery to lower pressure in the eye and prevent further damage to the optic nerve. Glaucoma affects people with both type 1 and type 2 diabetes. Your risk increases, however, the longer you've had diabetes, which may put people with type 1 diabetes since childhood at greater risk. Glaucoma generally has no early symptoms, so get screened annually. Medicare provides coverage for glaucoma screenings.

What you should know about cataracts

Cataracts are painless and are distinguished by a cloudy lens in the eye that may cause vision problems. Signs of a cataract include impaired distance vision, blurring of vision, decreased night vision, sensitivity to glare and bright light, a frequent need for a new eyeglasses prescription, seeing halos around lights, needing brighter lights to read by, and double vision. In people without diabetes, cataracts are almost exclusively a problem in those over the age of sixty and result from the normal stress of aging. However, the high blood sugar of diabetes accelerates the formation of cataracts, and many people with diabetes get them in their thirties or forties; diabetes raises the risk for cataracts by about 40 percent. I was fifty when my ophthalmologist told me I had the first sign of a slow-growing cataract.

Recommended treatment for a cataract is minor surgery whereby a small incision is made to the eye to remove the cloudy lens and an artificial lens is implanted. An annual eye exam is the best way to detect the beginning of a cataract, and keeping blood sugars as close to normal as possible is the best prevention. As with glaucoma, people who have diabetes are at risk for cataracts, and the risk is greater for those who have had diabetes longer.

What you should know about diabetic retinopathy

Of the three diabetes eye diseases, diabetic retinopathy is the most serious and the most common; it occurs in 90 percent of people with type 1 diabetes and in 65 percent of people with type 2 diabetes. It is estimated that between 40 and 45 percent of Americans with diabetes will have some stage of diabetic retinopathy. My friend Seth Bernstein, an optometrist, said that most people with diabetes may have retinopathy within five years of diagnosis as a result of uncontrolled blood sugars. These statistics sound awfully high, but neither Seth, who's had type 1 diabetes for almost twenty years, nor I, who have had it for thirty-seven years, have any retinopathy. The message: Don't let the risk profile get you down; get your blood sugars down instead. See your eye doctor every year, because diabetic retinopathy is one of the most preventable diabetic complications.

There are two types of diabetic retinopathy, nonproliferative and proliferative. Nonproliferative retinopathy is less severe; blood vessels in the retina weaken or swell and may leak fluid or become blocked from providing blood to the retina. Your vision is generally not affected and no treatment is necessary. To prevent progression of the disease, you should keep your blood sugar, blood pressure, and cholesterol levels as close to normal as possible.

In proliferative retinopathy the small blood vessels in the retina become severely damaged and close off completely, and new blood vessels grow. The new vessels are abnormal and fragile and tend to break, releasing blood into the eye. This causes your vision to blur or seem cloudy. You may see dark, floating spots. At its most severe, retinopathy can cause blindness. Hemorrhages, discharges of blood from the blood vessels, often happen and can even happen during sleep. Half of those people who have proliferative retinopathy also have macular edema, a condition wherein fluid leaks into the macula, which is the small and highly sensitive central area of the retina that is responsible for straight-ahead vision.

Tip to Make You Tops

Ocuvite®, an over-the-counter antioxidant, may help reduce the risk of developing macular problems. The Age-Related Eye Disease Study (AREDS) sponsored by the federal government's National Eye Institute followed 3,600 patients with varying stages of advanced macular degeneration (AMD) and found that antioxidants slow the progression of macula changes. They can also reduce the risk of developing AMD by about 25 percent.

If caught early, both nonproliferative and proliferative retinopathy can be treated, and significant damage can be avoided. Both proliferative retinopathy and macular edema are treated with laser surgery, which shrinks the abnormal and leaky blood vessels. Timely treatment can reduce the risk of blindness by 95 percent in people with proliferative retinopathy. Laser surgery can cause some loss of peripheral vision and can impair color and night vision, but laser treatment is very effective at saving the rest of your sight.

Joan, a religious studies teacher I met, told me that ever since she got diabetes more than fifty years ago at the age of thirteen, she has always prayed for two things: strength and courage. Joan's first diabetic complication was hemorrhaging of her eyes. "It was like taking a black magic marker, putting it in water, and rubbing it over my eyes. That's what I saw all day." After twenty-eight laser surgeries on both eyes, which did rob Joan of her color vision, her sight was saved. Owen, sixty-nine years old and a retired engineer, was diagnosed with type 2 diabetes at the age of forty-nine, while in the midst of a painful divorce. Owen ignored his diabetes the first ten years. When he developed retinopathy, Owen had an awakening. "This isn't going to get any worse," he said to himself. Laser treatments stopped Owen's retinopathy from progressing, and his eyesight is just fine today.

Get an annual dilated eye exam

Even though your general practitioner may look at your eyes during a routine visit, it's important to have your eyes checked annually by a specialist who can detect a serious eye problem. Eye diseases such as retinopathy typically don't cause any symptoms until a late stage of the disease. Even if you don't notice any vision problem, you should have a dilated eye exam every year to detect the beginning of any eye problem while it's early enough to prevent damage.

In a dilated eye exam, an eye specialist puts special drops in your eyes that cause your pupil (the center opening) to open wider so he or she can examine your retina, the area behind your eyes, for damaged nerve tissue and any changes to the blood vessels. The exam is painless, but take it from me—leaving your ophthalmologist's office on a sunny day without sunglasses is not! Come prepared, or your eyes will tear all the way home.

Tip to Make You Tops

Take the following steps to avoid eye problems:

- Keep your blood glucose in the target range your doctor has set.
- Control high blood pressure, maintain your proper weight, eat less salt, and, if necessary, take medication. Stress reducers such as yoga and biofeedback may help.
- Keep your cholesterol at acceptable levels—high cholesterol damages blood vessels.
- Don't smoke—smoking damages blood vessels.
- Get a dilated eye exam performed by an eye specialist once a year.

It's not safe for people with diabetes to exercise or play sports.

TRUTH: *Actually*, it is. But if you use insulin or a glucose-lowering medication, you need to know what precautions to take so your blood sugar doesn't go too low or too high.

Many people think you shouldn't exercise or play sports because if you use insulin or a medication that prompts your pancreas to produce insulin (such as Glucotrol®, Amaryl®, Glyburide®, Prandin®, or Starlix®), physical activity may cause hypo- or hyperglycemia. Also, Byetta® and Symlin®, can lower post-prandial (after a meal) blood glucose levels, especially when activity occurs shortly after a meal. The primary reason why your blood sugar may go too low is that physical exertion causes muscles to take up extra glucose (sugar) from the blood stream and allows insulin to work more efficiently; the combined effect can be too little sugar left in your blood.

Exercise usually lowers blood sugar. However, if your blood sugar is already high (over 300 mg/dl or 16.7 mmol/l) when you begin your activity and you don't have enough insulin to get the glucose from your blood stream into your cells, the cells will continue to send signals that they need glucose for fuel, and your liver will continue to create it. Glucose will then continue to build up in your blood, elevating your blood sugar levels even further. In addition, stress hormones are released during exercise, which causes the liver to send even more glucose into the blood. That having been said, it doesn't mean it's not safe to exercise or play sports. It means you need to follow some basic guidelines: Pay close attention to the balance among food, exercise, and medicine.

Outstanding athletes with diabetes prove you can safely work out and enjoy physical activity. Gary Hall, ten-time Olympic gold-medalist swimmer, was diagnosed with type 1 diabetes at the age of twenty-five. Already an Olympic medalist, Hall worked with his endocrinologist to learn how to manage his blood sugars and continues to swim competitively. At the Olympic competition following his diagnosis in 2000, he won a gold and a silver medal, setting a new American record for the fifty-meter freestyle.

Will Cross, who has lived with type 1 diabetes for more than thirty years, has climbed the highest mountain peaks on all seven continents and walked to the North and South Poles. In 2001 he climbed fifteen unmapped, unexplored mountains in Greenland.

David Weingard got type 1 diabetes seven years ago at age thirty-six but has since completed two Ironman triathlons (an ultra-endurance sport consisting of swimming, cycling, and running). After his diagnosis, Weingard spent a year simulating his swims and bike rides again and again, constantly measuring his blood sugars and logging his numbers in order to learn his body's response to exercise, food, and medicine. During one of his races, it rained all day, and his protected glucose meter on the handlebar of his bicycle broke. He could no longer test his blood sugar, but because he knew his body so well, he crossed the finish line in sixteen hours and eighteen minutes, making every cut-off time. Weingard's respect for training imparts a central message: No matter what level of physical activity you engage in, know your body.

You don't by any means have to be a professional athlete to exercise safely and accomplish great feats. At the 2005 Juvenile Diabetes Research Foundation's (JDRF) Children's Congress, 150 children aged three to seventeen participated in various activities; they hiked the Grand Canyon, skied, roller-skated, biked, river-rafted, and played varsity football. Some even won first place in competitive roller hockey, softball, karate, cross-country running, swimming, dirt biking, snowmobiling, and soccer, clearly demonstrating that exercise and diabetes are a safe and award-winning combination.

General guidelines to prevent hypoglycemia when physically active

If your blood sugar drops to 70 mg/dl (3.8 mmol/l) or below, this is called hypoglycemia and needs to be treated immediately. Symptoms of hypoglycemia include feeling faint, dizzy, weak, or confused; suffering a rapid heartbeat; shallow breathing; and irritability.

Always test before you begin—Check your blood sugar before you do any vigorous activity, whether running or yard work. If your blood sugar is under 100 mg/dl (5.5 mmol/l), eat some quick-acting carbohydrate before you exercise so that your blood sugar doesn't fall below 70 mg/dl (3.9 mmol/l). The amount of carbohydrate to ingest will depend on the intensity and duration of your activity. (Refer to Myth #30: When I feel the symptoms of low blood sugar, I should keep eating sweets until I feel better.)

Reduce your insulin—You can reduce the amount of insulin you take when you know you're going to be physically active. The dosage will depend on the vigorousness and duration of the planned activity. A diabetes educator can help you work out your dosing, or you can experiment by taking a little less insulin and testing your blood sugar before and after your activity.

Tweak your diet—Working with a dietitian, you can shift carbohydrates in your meal plan to ingest them just before you're active in order to fuel your exercise and maintain your blood sugar level. This may also mean you won't have to consume extra calories before an activity.

Strenuous activity can continue to affect blood sugar for as long as twelve to twenty-four hours, so test your blood sugar immediately after you finish your activity, a few hours after that, and a few hours after that to see that your blood sugar stays within your target range. Here are some safety measures you should also perform before or after you set out to be active:

- Always wear a diabetes ID bracelet.
- If you use insulin, inject into an area you use less when exercising, such as your abdomen rather than your legs or arms.
- Drink enough liquid before, during, and after your session. Being dehydrated can raise blood sugar.
- Always look your feet over for sores or blisters before and after you exercise.
- Carry glucose tablets, hard candy, or sweet snacks in case your blood sugar drops too low.

Tip to Make You Tops

An hour of housework can drop your blood sugar as much as an hour in the pool. Exercise physiologist Delaine Wright, who has diabetes, discovered she needed to make the same adjustment to her insulin dose for one hour of working in her yard as for one hour of kickboxing!

Preventing diabetic ketoacidosis

Physical activity while your blood sugar is high can raise your blood sugar even higher, which can put your body into a very dangerous state known as diabetic ketoacidosis (DKA). With insufficient insulin to transport sugar from the blood stream into the cells, the body begins to break down fat as an alternative energy source; the fat molecules produced are called ketones. A high incidence of ketones in the blood can be life-threatening.

DKA occurs almost exclusively in people with type 1 diabetes because they do not produce insulin, whereas most people with type 2, even if they take insulin injections, still produce enough insulin to transport some sugar from the blood stream into the cells. A small proportion of people with type 2 diabetes who have lost their own insulin production may also be susceptible to DKA.

Symptoms of ketoacidosis are an inability to keep anything down, rapid breathing, fruity breath, and feeling especially drowsy. My first diabetes interview was with Allison, a mature fourteen-year-old who got type 1 diabetes at age five. When I asked Allison, just to see what answer it might provoke, "Do you associate any smells with diabetes?" she immediately answered, "Roses! I don't like them anymore; when I have ketones I smell just like roses. Yuck, it's so grossly sweet!"

If your blood sugar is 300 mg/dl (16.7 mmol/l) or higher, perform a ketone test using a small kit you can purchase at the pharmacy. If your ketone test is positive, call your doctor right away and don't exercise. The ADA advises postponing any vigorous activity if you have ketones and beginning your activity only after you have brought your blood sugar down and it no longer shows ketones. ADA guidelines also say, however, that you don't have to avoid exercise on the basis of high blood sugar alone. If you feel fine, and a urine or ketone test shows you have no ketones, it's considered safe to exercise.

MYTH #38

Diabetes has nothing to do with erectile dysfunction or female sexual problems.

TRUTH: *Actually*, having diabetes can cause both of these problems, which affect about 50 percent of men and 25 percent of women with diabetes.

According to the National Institute of Diabetes and Digestive and Kidney Diseases (NIDDK), men with uncontrolled diabetes are three times more likely than men without diabetes to experience some erectile dysfunction (ED). In fact, ED is often what brings men to their doctor's office to then hear a diagnosis of diabetes. ED is defined as the inability to achieve and/or maintain an erection on at least half the occasions a man attempts to do so. Just as sustained high blood sugar can damage the nerves and small and large blood vessels throughout the body, they can damage the nerves and blood vessels leading to and within the penis. Some statistics say 50 percent of men with diabetes will experience ED within ten years of their diagnosis.

Women with diabetes are more susceptible than women without diabetes to have difficulty achieving orgasms; nerve damage within the vagina causes a gradual loss of sensation and sexual response. Women also report more discomfort during sexual intercourse; more frequent vaginal infections; and dryness, itching, or burning from prolonged high blood sugars. Janis Roszler, author of several books about diabetes and sex, says, "Women may experience sexually related symptoms even if they have good blood sugar control. Just having diabetes is now believed to be a trigger for sexual complications in women."

Contributing causes to erectile dysfunction

Cardiovascular disease, a complication of diabetes, can narrow or harden blood vessels, thus contributing to erectile problems; in men who suffer from both coronary artery disease (CAD) and diabetes, erectile dysfunction is nine times as likely to occur. Poor blood sugar control and smoking can also contribute by inhibiting the release of the chemical nitric oxide. Too little nitric oxide may hamper blood flow to the penis, which, again, makes it difficult to achieve or maintain an erection. Low testosterone is also a common cause of ED, and men who have diabetes are twice as likely as men who don't to have low testosterone levels. This condition is treatable, so check with your doctor. Certain medications, such as diuretics and beta blockers for blood pressure, and antidepressants, can also cause ED, as can depression.

Discuss your medications with your doctor and see whether they may be a factor in your ED, and if so, whether they can be changed. There are also prescription medications that may help alleviate ED. Viagra, Cialis, and Levitra all increase blood flow to the penis and make it easier to have and maintain an erection. Make sure your doctor knows all the medications you're taking, particularly nitrates to treat heart disease or alpha blockers to treat prostate enlargement or high blood pressure. There are also numerous other treatment options that increase blood flow to the penis, including vacuum pumps, constriction rings, injections, penile suppositories, penile support sleeves, and implants.

Tip to Make You Tops

The Mayo Clinic suggests the following additional ways to minimize the occurrence of, and treat, erectile dysfunction.

1. Control your blood sugar level. Good blood sugar control can prevent the nerve and blood vessel damage that leads to erectile dysfunction.
2. Limit your alcohol. Drinking more than two drinks a day can damage your blood vessels and make erectile dysfunction more likely.
3. Reduce stress. Stress can hamper erections.
4. Get physical. Regular exercise can keep your arteries clear and boost your stamina.
5. Fight fatigue. If you're well rested, you're less likely to struggle with erectile dysfunction.
6. Deal with anxiety and depression. Anxiety, depression, and the fear of having erectile problems can cause ED or make it worse.

Sexual complications for men as a result of diabetes aren't limited to erectile dysfunction. Men can also suffer decreased libido due to blood sugar swings, and, as diabetes educator Roszler points out, sexual distress. "Sex is a part of our identity, and performance anxiety can bring tension into a relationship. Further, a man's ability to feel sexual may also be compromised by weight gain and injection bruising." Seeing a therapist may help, along with any other treatments.

Sexual dysfunction in women

The extent of sexual dysfunction in women with diabetes has been explored less than in men. However, poor blood circulation and diabetes-related nerve damage are known to interfere with the ability of the vaginal area to become engorged with blood and lubricate upon arousal, compromising a woman's ability to enjoy sexual activity. Women may experience the inability to become or remain aroused. They may also lack sensation or the capacity to reach orgasm. It is also possible that women may have problems with arousal similar to those that confront men; just as the penis fails to become erect in a man, the clitoris in a woman may not respond to stimulation. As many as 35 percent of women with diabetes may experience little to no sexual response. A number of women with poorly controlled diabetes also suffer from urinary tract infections that can make sex painful and cause itching or burning.

Prescription or over-the-counter vaginal lubricant creams such as KY jelly may be effective for treating a variety of conditions that cause minor vaginal discomfort, including dryness. However, if these are not effective, discuss with your health care provider other options, such as hormone suppositories and Viagra (which some women use to enhance libido).

There may be multiple ramifications for women when sexual problems occur. A woman may fear intercourse if she has had pain in the past, and that stress may affect her blood sugar. The demands of diabetes (over and above being caretaker for the family or breadwinner if she plays these roles) may bring tension into her relationship, says sex expert Roszler, that decreases her interest in and energy for sex. A woman may worry about becoming pregnant, knowing it is unwise if her diabetes is not well controlled. She may also, like men, feel low self-esteem from diabetes-related weight gain and injection bruising. Because there is no medication for women that's been proven to stoke or sustain sexual desire and performance, and because the brain is the largest sexual organ in the body and most women connect emotionally, Roszler offers these suggestions to help a woman feel more sexual:

- If you're on a medication that's affecting your libido, try a different medication.
- Try self-stimulation, which can help your body lubricate and become aroused, and thus help you reconnect with enjoying sex.
- Participate in weekly dates with your partner, and get to know each other again away from everyday stresses.
- Schedule intimacy and lovemaking so that you have enough time to become aroused.
- Seek help if sad feelings are getting in the way of living your normal life.

Just as for men, taking steps to improve overall health may also help with some sexual problems: Make an extra effort to participate in some form of physical activity most days of the week. Follow a well-balanced meal plan that helps you achieve and maintain a healthful weight. Keep your blood sugar, blood pressure, and cholesterol in a healthful range. Reduce daily stress by adjusting your hectic schedule and participate in stress-reducing activities such as yoga, meditation, or chatting with friends. Limit your alcohol intake and don't smoke.

MYTH #39

There's nothing to help the pain in my feet!

TRUTH: *Actually*, there are several ways to reduce diabetic foot pain, including medication, relaxation techniques, herbal supplements, and exercise.

Medications are one approach to resolving diabetic foot pain generally caused by nerve damage (peripheral neuropathy), and your doctor may prescribe Lyrica® or Cymbalta®. Pain blockers, which include some antidepressants and antiseizure medications, are also used for diabetic foot pain. They can treat foot pain successfully, but you may have to use them for a few months before you know whether they'll work for you, and there can be a risk of side effects. Luckily, in addition to medication, there are several other ways to get relief from the sensitivity, numbness, tingling, or stabbing pain you may experience.

Many therapies, from simple walking to alternative treatments, can offer relief from foot pain. Nightly massaging a diabetic foot cream such as DiabetiDerm Foot Rejuvenating Cream into your feet rehydrates dry skin, softens calluses, smoothes irritated areas, and provides soothing warmth. Doing specific foot exercises and daily walking are excellent ways to help relieve pain; they both strengthen the muscles and ligaments in your feet and increase blood flow to your feet. Here's a simple foot exercise if you're just beginning: With your hands placed on a wall for support, rise up on your toes with both feet. Hold this position for five to ten seconds and then lower yourself slowly. Do this a few times as is comfortable, and work up to ten and then twenty repetitions. A more playful exercise is to see whether, while steadying yourself against a wall or the back of a chair, you can pick up a marble with your toes. Work up to ten repetitions.

Birgitta Rice, diabetes educator and foot specialist, advocates walking for anyone who can do it. Rice also recommends alternative treatments she's found effective for patients; she explains that both relaxation and visualization techniques and energy modalities such as acupressure and reflexology can stimulate greater blood flow to the feet, providing warmth and healing energy. Transcutaneous electrical nerve stimulation (TENS), which sends electrical current through the skin to block pain signals, and monochromatic infrared energy therapy, which increases blood flow to your feet, can also help relieve pain. Many patients find acupuncture, shiatsu, massage, and chiropractic treatments useful. And if all else fails, Rice says that surgery can provide effective pain relief.

Biofeedback has also proved very effective for alleviating foot pain. Rice was part of a randomized twelve-week study at the University of Wisconsin in Madison, where patients who had had painful foot ulcers for at least eight weeks and no more than two years were asked to visualize warming their feet through a standardized relaxation and biofeedback therapy called WarmFeet®. The technique is really quite simple, said Rice, who helped create it and uses it herself. Relaxation allows the arteries and capillaries of your peripheral blood vessels to dilate, so more blood flows through them to places such as your feet, bringing each foot additional oxygen, nutrients, and gentle warmth. This both prompts healing and relieves pain. Remarkably, not only did the participants get relief from their pain, but fourteen of the sixteen patients who used the relaxation technique completely healed their foot ulcers. For more information about WarmFeet®, contact Health Education for Life at 7412 Park View Drive, St. Paul, Minnesota 55112, or go online to www.WarmFeetKit.com.

> While at an American Diabetes Association Expo, foot specialist Birgitta Rice caught her shoe in the ribs of the escalator she was running up. She fell and the steel ribbing of the step pierced into her shin, leaving her with a half-inch-square wound bleeding ferociously. Rice cleaned her wound in the ladies bathroom and left for home so she could get off her foot right away. After applying triple antibiotic cream to the wound, Rice practiced the WarmFeet® technique several times during the next few days, experiencing a significant reduction in her pain. On the third day, not only was she pain-free but the sore was completely healed.

A powerhouse antioxidant—alpha lipoic acid

Since 1959 physicians in Germany have treated diabetic neuropathy with alpha lipoic acid, and it is widely used in Europe today to also prevent diabetes-related cataracts and macular degeneration. In 2003 a large collaborative study between the Mayo Clinic in Rochester, Minnesota, and the Russian Medical Academy for Advanced Studies in Moscow followed 120 patients, aged eighteen to seventy-four, in a double-blind study (that is, neither patients nor investigators knew which patients received ALA and which received a placebo). Findings showed that treatment with ALA improved nerve function and significantly and rapidly reduced the frequency and severity of neuropathy symptoms: tingling, numbness, burning, freezing, and extreme sensitivity to touch.

No harmful side effects have thus far been found with the recommended 600-mg/day use of ALA, and a four-year clinical trial is currently under way in the United States and Europe to continue studying the antioxidant. Also, a time-release formula is in development that may further improve ALA's efficiency.

Tip to Make You Tops

Under the direction of a diabetes educator, I took the antioxidant alpha lipoic acid (ALA) when I was experiencing, more often than usual, the intermittent tingling (a symptom of neuropathy) that I've been getting in one calf for more than twenty-five years. I took 600 mg daily, and within weeks the tingling decreased noticeably and was less persistent.

Depending on your age and the condition of your feet, surgery can also be an option for pain relief. Several surgical procedures relieve pressure on the nerves in your feet by opening the small tunnels through which the nerves pass and allowing more blood flow, which can reduce or relieve pain, tingling, and numbness.

Numerous pain relief therapies and techniques can help you alleviate foot pain, but keeping your blood sugars and your diabetes in good control is a pain-saving technique we can all use all the time. While researching this myth, I read online the story of a woman in her late twenties who had changed her unhealthful lifestyle habits four years earlier, after living with diabetes for almost fifteen years. One of the first things she noticed was a marked improvement of the neuropathy in her feet. In response to her story, forty-one people with diabetes posted comments within hours, and this one typifies what many said: "I have a long history of type 1 diabetes, sixty years. I had very painful neuropathy in both of my feet. In 2000, I went on a pump and since then have much tighter control. My A1C now ranges from 5.7 percent to 6.5 percent. After the first two years of my lower A1C, I lost all the pain from neuropathy in my feet. I am sure tight control is the reason."

MYTH #40

Diabetes certainly doesn't affect my teeth or gums.

TRUTH: *Actually,* diabetes can put you at greater risk for gum disease, mouth infections, and possibly cavities.

Janet was eight years old when she got type 1 diabetes; unfortunately, she didn't get the necessary education to help her manage it. By the time she was twenty she'd already suffered multiple diabetic complications, but it was being fitted for dentures—top and bottom—that motivated her to start taking care of her diabetes. "Because my sugar had been so high for so long, it rotted all my teeth. Sitting in that dentist's chair, I was thinking, 'I'm twenty-six years old and I'm dealing with something old people get.' I'd had dreams all my life about my teeth falling out, and here it was happening, they were pulling out all my teeth. That was my wake-up call."

Although Janet's story is extreme, Jean Bertschart Roemer, diabetes educator and pediatric nurse practitioner, says it illustrates how serious the risk of periodontal (gum) disease can be with poorly controlled diabetes. Roemer has followed children with diabetes from diagnosis to their early twenties, witnessing how gum and mouth infections occur more frequently in people with diabetes, particularly when blood sugars are consistently high.

At the 2008 ADA Scientific Conference, oral health was a new and hot topic. "One of the many complications of diabetes is a greater risk for periodontal disease," said Maria E. Ryan, DDS, PhD, professor of oral biology and pathology, and director of clinical research for the School of Dental Medicine at Stony Brook University in New York. Persistent high glucose levels in the blood contribute to the destruction of bone and gum tissue, said Dr. George W. Taylor, associate professor of dentistry at the University of Michigan's Schools of Dentistry and Public Health.

Elevated blood glucose levels raise the risk of infection everywhere in your body, including your mouth. Periodontal disease is an infection and chronic inflammation of the tissues surrounding and supporting the teeth. It is a major cause of tooth loss in adults. In periodontitis, plaque hardens into calculus (tartar), gums gradually begin to pull away from the teeth, and pockets form between the teeth and gums. Awful as this may sound, people often do not know they have periodontal disease because it is usually painless. Robert Eber, DDS, clinical professor of periodontics and oral medicine at the University of Michigan, opened my eyes to the seriousness of periodontal disease when he confirmed that, yes, "size matters." "In periodontal disease, the total surface area of inflamed soft tissue surrounding a tooth is about the same surface area as the palm of one's hand," said Eber. "Imagine if you had an ulcerated, inflamed area that size on your leg. You wouldn't leave that untreated."

High blood sugars slow the healing process, so mouth infections are harder to treat or eliminate, worsening periodontal disease. At the same time, periodontal disease worsens glycemic control. The body reacts to gum disease with inflammation, which raises blood sugar and can increase insulin resistance. Dr. Taylor cited several recent studies at the ADA Conference that confirm not only the link between periodontal disease and high blood sugars but also between gum disease and other diabetes complications.

Although periodontal disease makes diabetes worse, it also appears that periodontal treatment can bring about a reduction in the risk for diabetes complications.

Signs of periodontal disease

The first sign of gum disease is often sore, swollen, or red gums that bleed when you brush your teeth or floss. As infection advances, your gums may pull away from your teeth. A more severe infection is marked by spots between your teeth and gums that are filled with pus. Pain in your mouth or sinuses, discoloration of your teeth, and tooth sensitivity to heat and cold can also be markers of an infection. If you notice any of these signs or the ones below, you should get to your dentist immediately.

- Bad breath
- Loose teeth
- Teeth that are moving away from each other
- A change in the way your teeth fit together when you bite
- A change in the way your dentures fit

Mouth infections can be painful and can make chewing painful. They can also cause dry mouth, which can foster the growth of

---

Tip to Make You Tops

Babies who are given bottles in their crib to keep their blood sugar up, with no chance to brush afterward, are susceptible to what's called "baby-bottle mouth," which can lead to cavities. Give your baby water after a bottle to rinse his or her mouth.

bacteria that promote cavities and enamel loss. Mouth infections can also cause fungal yeast infections called candida. Candida look like white, curd-like patches that easily scrape off your tongue and leave a red, ulcerated area underneath. Dayna, who got type 2 diabetes at the age of sixteen, said that her most hateful complications were both the mouth infections that ate away at the enamel between her teeth and a mouth full of cavities. "I never had a cavity until I got diabetes, ever," said Dayna.

Hidden infections that can affect your gums and jawbone

Infections that affect dental structures, including infections that affect root canals, gums, and jawbones, are some of the most common types of hidden infections. Among the things your dentist should do to examine your gums very carefully is to tap every tooth to see whether one or more is tender. If your dentist does find a problem, he or she may need to refer you to an endodontist, who deals with root canals and the jawbone, or a periodontist, who treats infected gums.

Tip to Make You Tops

Dr. Richard Bernstein cautions that unexplained high blood sugars can indicate a gum infection. If a patient calls his office and complains of a recent onset of high blood sugars but has no signs of illness, Dr. Bernstein first asks that patient whether he or she is reusing insulin syringes, which can contaminate insulin and render it less effective. If not, Dr. Bernstein recommends his patient get to the dentist immediately to determine whether there is an oral infection.

Jean Betschart Roemer, Pediatric Nurse Practitioner and Certified Diabetes Educator

Five Ways to Take Care of Your Diabetes

1. Expect that you can't manage your blood sugars perfectly, but if they're usually not in your target range, take small steps to improve them.
2. Take care of your diabetes routinely so you have less of the extreme high and low blood sugars that will prevent you from doing the things you want to do.
3. Work out a "survival mode" plan of care—one that entails the minimum amount of work to manage your diabetes so that you can fall back on it when times are stressful. "Musts" on your plan are checking your blood glucose and taking your medication.
4. Do whatever it takes to get your blood glucose control to be the best it can be. If you see a product advertised and wonder whether you can try it, ask your doctor. Sometimes you will hit upon a product, medication, schedule adjustment, or habit that works better than your current treatment plan.
5. Advocate for yourself and for the best diabetes care. Seek out diabetes educators, dietitians, and physicians who are experienced in diabetes care. Don't settle for just doing OK!

How to best prevent gum infections and other oral hygiene problems

The ways in which you can protect yourself from infection include brushing your teeth at least twice daily and flossing every day. If your teeth are too tightly spaced for flossing, you can find various dental cleaning tools in your pharmacy specially designed to help clean your teeth and gums. Just as with babies, if you treat a blood sugar low in the middle of the night, rinse your mouth afterward with water to wash away the sugar. If your teeth and gums are healthy, see your dentist every six months for a check-up and cleaning. Finally, make sure your dentist knows you have diabetes, and remind him or her at your visit. You want your dentist watching for signs of gum and mouth disease right along with you.

Psych Myths

MYTH #41

I can't ever take a break from dealing with my diabetes.

TRUTH: *Actually,* not only *can* you take a break, it's highly recommended.

Dr. William Polonsky, founder of the Behavioral Diabetes Institute, says not only *can* you take a break from diabetes, you *must*. While attending a diabetes conference, Polonsky told me, diabetes educators were adding up all the tasks involved in managing diabetes, and they stopped counting when they reached 150! "Periodic mini-vacations from the demands of diabetes," says Polonsky, "are required. They keep you mentally healthy and keep you going."

A survey Polonsky designed and conducts regularly with patients, called the Diabetes Distress Scale survey, reveals that patients' greatest frustration with diabetes is the enormity of it all. *How do I stay on this diet? I have no time for regular exercise! I'm sixty-six and now I've got to go to the gym? How am I going to test my blood sugar so many times? Do I really have to take so many pills? You want me to take shots every day?! When do I get a break?* In fact, Polonsky was shocked when he learned patients actually welcomed a week's stay at the Joslin Diabetes Clinic. "It was a huge relief to people to spend a week where *they* didn't have to take responsibility for, or be in charge of, their diabetes. The dirty little secret," says Polonsky, "is everybody takes vacations from diabetes because no one can do diabetes perfectly all the time." What's important is taking a "safe" vacation and making sure you come back from your vacation.

Taking breaks from your diabetes management helps you restore your energy and let go of stress, and it helps everyone around you; they benefit from your being less stressed. Parents of children with diabetes may think they can't ever take a break, but diabetes educator Betty Brackenridge says it's vital, and in her book *Draw Wide the Circle of Love*, she explains various ways to do so. One is to develop a support circle of extended family members and good friends who can pitch in by teaching them about diabetes and how to do blood sugar checks. This not only lets you take a break but also keeps grandmas and grandpas close. A pediatric endocrinologist instructs his young patients and their parents to take two days off a month from testing blood sugars, provided it isn't two days in a row and an adult is present.

Tips for taking a "safe" vacation

- Create a plan with your health care team so that your diabetes control isn't compromised. For instance, learn ahead of time how to adjust your medications for any circumstance that may arise.
- Understand that you're not quitting your diabetes care altogether, just taking a very brief break. For example, you might take one night off a week from your diabetes-friendly meal plan.
- Skip a noncritical blood glucose check once or twice a week.
- Check your blood sugar less often one day a week when you tend to eat and exercise the way you usually do and so

have confidence that you can safely guesstimate how you're doing.

Paul, a successful businessman, takes a diabetes holiday every Friday night. "My wife and I have family over and we put out cheeses, pepperoni, and antipasto, and I eat and drink whatever I want and cover it with my insulin. For four hours I'm no longer 'diabetic' in my mind; I'm just a regular guy. I think it's better to maintain good control six days a week and live a little one night a week for a few hours than to have poor control much of the time." Larry, who's seventy-six and has had type 2 diabetes for thirty-five years, "goes crazy" with food on infrequent occasions. "The brilliant endocrinologist that I see," Larry told me, "agreed to this approach years ago." Lara, who's had type 1 diabetes for thirty-three years, says, "I skip a meal if I'm not hungry. I check my blood sugar to make sure I'm OK and then just go on about my business." It sounds silly that this is a vacation for Lara, but for more than two decades she had to eat to prevent lows.

Having someone help share the load can also be a vacation

Asking someone to help you with a diabetes-related task can take a lot of stress off your shoulders. Maybe a family member or friend will do the grocery shopping or cooking for a few days. I know a man who tests his wife's blood sugar for her when she's tired. He gets her meter and lancing device, takes the test strip out of the vial, puts it into the machine, pricks her finger for her and waits for the reading, giving her a break and much needed support. One woman gave her sister the best wedding gift possible. On the day of the wedding she said to her sister, the bride, "Just stick out your finger when you need to know your blood sugar, and I'll do the rest."

Maybe your spouse can accompany you on a walk after a meal to make walking more enjoyable. Who knows? It may become a regular habit. Maybe your partner or a good friend will just be an active listener so you can express your fears or concerns when diabetes feels like too much. Sometimes our loved ones are just waiting for us to ask for their help; they want to give it but just don't know how.

Tip to Make You Tops

When I got married eight years ago, my husband would stand over my meter as I did my morning blood sugar check. I was appalled. Having him there made me uncomfortable—what if a "bad" number came up? I'd feel embarrassed and ashamed, so I chased him away. It didn't take long for me to realize that this was neither a good way to start a marriage nor a good way to handle my diabetes, so I let him watch. I used the time to educate him about diabetes, and I shared my feelings about living with diabetes. After about six blood sugar checks, he understood much better what I deal with on a daily basis and asked what he could do that would truly help me.

Now this somewhat shy and conservative Dutch man asks the waitress when we're out to dinner whether the chef will substitute a green vegetable for the rice or potatoes, just as he's seen me do. But I was never so touched as one day when, as we left the house, I saw him put into *his* pocket the little rolls of Swee-Tarts I carry in case my blood sugar drops, so he could protect me if needed.

Recognizing unsafe vacations from diabetes

Unsafe vacations are those breaks from managing your diabetes that you rarely plan for, that go on for a long period of time, or that render you faithful to part of your management but not to another (for example, you take your medications regularly but never test your blood sugar). Dr. Polonsky is quick to say that if you find yourself taking "unsafe" vacations from diabetes, this may mean either that you need to develop a more practical diabetes plan with your health care provider or that you may be experiencing emotional issues that are causing burnout or depression. Most of us can feel this way from time to time—psychologist Polonsky discovered that close to 70 percent of people with diabetes feel an underlying sense of dread fearing long-term complications.

One of the fastest remedies when you're feeling down is to get accurate information that will help you to take care of your diabetes and to realize it's worth the effort. However, if you think you may be depressed or if loved ones are telling you so, seek help. Seeking help from a counselor, therapist, or religious leader also isn't just for extreme times and rare cases; rather, as a diabetes psychologist said to me, it is a natural adjunct to good diabetes management.

"Without a doubt you will most likely live a long and healthy life with diabetes," says Polonsky, "if you take care of it, and part of taking care of diabetes is to remember that safe breaks now and then are a necessary, allowable part of your treatment plan."

If my doctor says it's time for me to take insulin, I'm a failure.

TRUTH: *Actually,* if your doctor says it's time for you to take insulin, it's only because that's the best way to manage your blood sugar.

The primary goal of diabetes treatment is to keep blood sugars as close to normal as possible to reduce the risk of diabetic complications. Toward that end, most people with type 2 diabetes begin a treatment program of diet, exercise, and perhaps one glucose-lowering pill. Then, within a few years, either the dose or the amount of pills they take (or both) is increased. Also, insulin may be added to their protocol.

The truth is this: If you control your blood sugar as close to normal as possible, along with the other conditions of diabetes such as high cholesterol, high triglycerides, and high blood pressure, and if you lose weight if necessary and get regular exercise, you have the greatest opportunity to stabilize your diabetes and slow or perhaps even halt its progress. You also may be able to eliminate the need for medication (although the need for medication may return). But this doesn't mean that if you are prescribed insulin, you are a failure.

Even if you do "all the right things" to take care of your diabetes, you might at some point need insulin. How the body responds to diabetes is highly individualized, and for some people genetics, certain medicines, and other health conditions are also determinants of how their diabetes will progress.

What's also true is this: Judging yourself a failure if you need to use insulin is just that—a judgment—and it's one that is not in your best interest. Psychologists say it will benefit you much more to understand that if insulin is being recommended, it's simply because insulin is the best medicine to manage your diabetes. Now it's up to you to commit to or continue to do your best to manage your diabetes, to respect yourself for your efforts, and to move forward. The only "failure" related to using insulin occurs if your doctor is telling you to do so and you refuse.

Tip to Make You Tops

Failure is not a useful or accurate way to view insulin being added to your treatment plan, says clinical psychologist Wendy Satin-Rapaport. "The best way to see insulin is, 'Aren't I lucky there is something available that will help me control my blood sugar so well that I can have the quality of life I want and deserve?!'"

"Insulin changed my life," says Gary, having used it for five years. "I have so much more energy, and my blood sugars are in such good control. I only wish I hadn't fought my doctor for so long." Gary began his treatment on oral medication, a healthful diet, and exercise, and this kept his diabetes in reasonably good control, with A1C values around 7.0 percent, for the first few years. "But then my glucose readings started increasing and becoming unpredictable," Gary said. "After five years of treatment, my doctor and my wife suggested that I start using insulin to improve my diabetes management. I was dead set against it. I was afraid to give myself injections, I didn't want to begin what I saw as a lifetime dependency, and I thought I had failed somehow. It wasn't until I became a speaker, talking to fellow patients about better control, that it dawned on me that *everyone* is dependent on insulin; it's just that people with type 1 diabetes and many people with type 2 diabetes need lab-made insulin to augment the lesser amounts their bodies are producing."

Still reluctant, Gary waited another year to start insulin, until his blood sugar jumped to above 200 mg/dl (11.1 mmol/L) and wouldn't come down. Always slim, he dropped from 135 pounds to 110 pounds, and fatigue forced him to give up his love of travel. Within two days of his starting a basal (long-acting) insulin, Gary's blood sugar dropped significantly, his energy returned, his mood brightened, and he scheduled his first adventure trip in a long time.

Why do we feel like a failure when insulin is introduced?

Psychologist Wendy Satin-Rapaport says one reason why people associate insulin with failure is that it seems to be the last straw after so many "failures" with diabetes tasks: years of unsuccessful attempts to lose weight, not being able to adhere to an exercise regimen, or getting a complication that they've worked so hard to avoid.

People with diabetes may also experience "diabetes aggravation," uncomfortable feelings brought on by situations unique to the process of living with diabetes. Repeatedly experiencing these situations heightens feelings of failure. Such situations include

- Health worries about the present and future
- Anxieties and frustrations related to blood sugar testing
- Criticism from family members or one's medical team
- Food temptations at mealtimes and parties

Steps to counteract distress and maximize your power

One way to address and transform feelings of failure is through a process called self-inquiry. Self-inquiry involves paying attention to your "internal dialogue": what you tell yourself. Listen to the thoughts streaming through your head about diabetes, and ask yourself questions about any feelings of failure. Then try to uncover what thoughts and beliefs are creating them. For example, if your blood sugar is 300 mg/dl (16.7 mmol/l), you might be telling yourself, "I'm not testing anymore. I'm no good at it!" Instead, look at the situation objectively and take the blame away: "Hmmm . . . my blood sugar is 300 mg/dl (16.7 mmol/l). How might that have happened? I will give myself some insulin and test in two hours. The number will go down, and I'll feel good having handled the situation."

Also, how you view diabetes can help you overcome feelings of failure.

- See some of the problems that diabetes presents as similar to what other people without diabetes face as they age. This helps lessen feelings of isolation and resentment.

- Let go of fear and "It's not fair!" Instead focus on what you love, what gives you pleasure, and what you're grateful for and appreciate.
- Explore why you put off your health tasks or quit too quickly. Perfectionism? Fear of change? Anger? Anxiety? Social self-consciousness?
- Recognize your successes managing diabetes and the things you do well. This will help keep you motivated.

Tip to Make You Tops

Succeeding with your management tasks helps you feel empowered and overcomes feelings of failure. These steps may help:

- *Monitor your actions*—For example, create a food diary and look for patterns.
- *Enlist stimulus control*—Leave exercise clothes where you will see them as a cue.
- *Visualize success*—See yourself smiling while looking at normal blood sugars on your meter.
- *Engage in stress management*—Ask for support, learn a relaxation technique such as yoga or meditation, think positively, and see the humor in situations.
- *Schedule regular doctor appointments*—Even when you have nothing to report, regular visits help you stay motivated and moving.
- *Concentrate on improvement*—Pick one task you can improve by breaking it down into small, specific, manageable steps.

- Watch out for negative or catastrophic thinking, and change it into forgiving, realistic, and optimistic thoughts that lead to more competent behaviors.

While you are living with diabetes, there will be times when you lapse, relapse, collapse, and deviate from good management. But you will keep feelings of failure at bay by seeing the successful results of your efforts, remembering you can positively affect your life, knowing you can exert control over your diabetes, and remaining hopeful.

I should be able to take diabetes in stride.

TRUTH: *Actually,* it's nearly impossible to manage everything diabetes requires without feeling frustrated, angry, or blue at times.

Living with diabetes is demanding, and it's bound to create stress at times. To begin with, the bulk of responsibility lies on your shoulders to take care of yourself and perform the many tasks diabetes requires: watching what you eat and balancing your food and medicine daily; testing and logging your blood sugars; finding time for exercise; scheduling and keeping doctor appointments; refilling prescriptions; going for lab tests; dealing with sick days and slogging through days when high blood sugars make you feel slow as molasses; not to mention managing your family, work, and other life responsibilities.

Then there are the emotional stresses and strains of diabetes: concern about complications and your future, feeling guilty if you're not managing everything as well as you might, feeling as though you're "cheating" on your diet, or constantly asking, "Why me?" You may feel embarrassed if you have to take an injection or treat low blood sugar in public, and you may feel discomfort telling your hostess, "I'm sorry, I can't eat that beautiful seven-layer cake you slaved over all day." Plus, you have to deal with family members who, albeit out of love, always seem to be telling you what you should and shouldn't eat and do.

How to take diabetes more in stride

No one can always take diabetes in stride. Rather, psychologists offer these tips:

- Focus on being proud of your efforts, even when the outcome isn't what you'd hoped it would be. With diabetes, you cannot always control the outcome.
- Give yourself a day off now and then to recharge your energy. We all need occasional breaks from diabetes, just as we need breaks from our jobs to rest and recharge.
- Become more realistic in your expectations: Know that diabetes is hard work, and it is not realistic or helpful to think you won't have days when you feel overwhelmed, sad, or stressed.
- Give yourself a pat on the back for the time you spend attempting to control diabetes, and consider it time well spent.
- Pace yourself. You are in this for the long haul, so don't sweat the small stuff.

Tip to Make You Tops

The Behavioral Diabetes Institute offers free seminars to help people deal with the emotions of living with diabetes. Check its Web site, www.behavioraldiabetes.org, or call 858-336-8693. You can also download the institute's brochure "The Emotional Side of Diabetes: 10 Things You Need to Know" to help you manage diabetes with more ease.

Patients' top challenges and how to deal with them

Struggling with diabetes from time to time is so normal that diabetes clinicians and psychologists came up with this list of patients' five top stressors. Luckily, they also came up with ways to help defuse them.

1. *Challenge: The exasperating stuff other people say.* This is patients' number-one gripe. "You got diabetes because you're fat!" and "You can't eat that!" are just two of the exasperating things patients often hear.

   What to do: Recognize that most people are concerned about your welfare and don't know how to help. Tell them, "I know you're trying to be helpful, but saying that doesn't really help me." Then let people know what they *can* do that will help you.

2. *Challenge: Feeling alone with your diabetes.* Most people with diabetes feel isolated and alone much of the time.

   What to do: Reach out to a friend, or find others with diabetes with whom you can share your feelings. Join a diabetes support group or enroll in a class or seminar. Online message boards, forums, and Web blogs allow you to connect with others over the Internet. Be a "diabetes buddy" with someone, and keep each other motivated.

3. *Challenge: Never feeling like you get a break.* Patients report that it's often the enormity of it all and the constant effort that are overwhelming.

   What to do: Give yourself a "diabetes vacation" now and then. It's OK to check your glucose less often one day, skip a workout at the gym for a great night out with friends, or eat a few foods you don't usually allow yourself. Turn off the guilt-o-meter and let yourself enjoy. (For further information about diabetes vacations, see Myth #41: I can't ever take a break from dealing with my diabetes.)

4. *Challenge: Feeling like you have to do it all perfectly.* It's just not possible to do diabetes perfectly, and furthermore it's not necessary.

   What to do: Know that good management is doable. Set targets for your care, and appreciate each step you take toward those targets.

5. *Challenge: The expense of diabetes.* Diabetes medicines, supplies, and education can be costly.

   What to do: If you have health insurance, find out whether your plan covers a mail-order pharmacy; these offer supplies with a lower co-pay. Investigate which government and pharmaceutical agencies offer free or low-cost supplies. (For further information on cutting expenses, see Myth #46: Financial help for diabetes treatment, supplies, and support services is not available to me.)

Clinical psychologist Susan Guzman of the Behavioral Diabetes Institute, says, "You can't do diabetes perfectly nor should you try.

Tip to Make You Tops

If you're picking up your supplies at a local pharmacy, ask your doctor to help you synchronize the prescriptions so that you have only one pickup per month. At home, keep your supplies all in one place where it's easy to see how much you have left, and before you run out, mark on a calendar when it will be time to refill prescriptions.

That only sets you up for failure because it's not realistic." Instead, Guzman advises, realize that "good enough is fine" when it comes to diabetes management and to prevent or delay complications, and that you are capable of managing your diabetes "good enough."

Patients share their coping methods

In addition to the medical experts' solutions, here are pearls of wisdom from fellow patients about what they do when diabetes feels like too much. Larry, a doctor and researcher, seals himself away in his workshop designing and making pens. Another friend admits that sex works pretty well to put a smile back on his face. Tim's sanity check is taking his blood sugar reading to see whether a high or a low blood sugar is causing his mood. If his blood sugar is around 100, he laughs out loud and is immediately cheered. Stephan, a former military man, finds release writing down his feelings in a journal. Carolyn, the most cheerful eighty-year-old woman I know, goes to her local swimming pool and floats in the water where her cares "just float away." As for me, shedding a few tears and then pouring my heart out to my attentive husband work wonders.

Here are more ways in which fellow patients cope:

- "Reach out to friends or my spouse for a heart-to-heart talk."
- "Throw on my sweat suit and start doing something that makes me sweat."
- "Do something I enjoy, like slip into a hot bath, go for a walk, or sit in my lounge chair and listen to classical music while sipping a glass of wine."

- "Do something relaxing like take a yoga class."
- "Do something distracting like go to a movie, pick up a good book, or plan my next vacation."
- "Talk to myself, saying, 'It will be better tomorrow.'"
- "Give it to God and let Him help shoulder it."

"In the end, to keep yourself going," says Dr. William Polonsky, "you have to have hope that it's possible to live a long and healthy life with diabetes, and with all the research, now we know this is true." Taking diabetes in stride means knowing there will be tough times and knowing you'll get through them.

LOOKING THROUGH THE LENS OF . . .
William Polonsky, Associate Clinical Professor in Psychiatry at the University of California, San Diego, and Certified Diabetes Educator

Five Ways to Take Care of Your Diabetes

1. Don't do diabetes alone. Having someone supporting your efforts will make you more successful.
2. Know your test results. Knowing what they mean and what to do about them can free you of unnecessary worry.
3. Be kind to yourself. Have some clear, reachable goals, not goals that are unnecessary and unachievable.
4. Have a plan. Know where to concentrate your efforts to get more bang for your buck.
5. Harness your environment. If your treadmill is under the couch, you won't benefit much. Set up your tasks in a way that works for you.

MYTH #44

Teens take better care of themselves when they understand the importance of doing so.

TRUTH: *Actually*, understanding doesn't make teens more responsible. Making them accountable for their behavior does.

Most parents believe that if their teen understands the consequences of not taking care of his diabetes, he will act more responsibly. But that's not true, says Joe Solowiejczyk, a family therapist and diabetes nurse who's been helping parents for more than twenty years develop in their children greater responsibility for managing their diabetes. "Don't get me wrong," says Solowiejczyk, "Kids are smart, very smart. But simply instilling *understanding* is not the way to get them to change poor behavior." Treating your teen's irresponsible approach to diabetes management in the same way as any other irresponsible behavior and applying the same consequences, such as withholding videogames or other privileges, makes your teen more responsible managing his or her diabetes.

Parents want to do everything possible to protect their child or make allowances, says Solowiejczyk. Their child has already been punished enough just by having diabetes. "But parents in my workshop always nod their heads when I say, 'If you're a worried parent now, you won't be able to stand it when your teen heads off to college and you don't trust that he can take care of himself. It's your job to apply consequences now to save your child from consequences later."

Clinicians agree that classes, support groups, and summer camps may help teenagers feel good about themselves. However, their attempts to use "understanding the consequences of poor diabetes care" as a motivational tactic rarely produce change in behavior. Last year at the American Association of Diabetes Educators conference, I sat in on a presentation about adolescent development and diabetes self-care. I learned that adolescents are only beginning to master sophisticated thinking, such as seeing the links among their decisions, their actions, and the results. Indeed, it isn't until our early twenties that this type of cognitive thinking is fully developed.

Clinical psychologist Wendy Satin-Rapaport, who has worked with families for thirty years, says that "understanding" as a general theoretical concept (for example, your child *understanding* that if he doesn't test his blood sugar multiple times a day now, he may get complications fifteen years from now) doesn't motivate his behavior. But parents *understanding* why their child makes certain choices (for instance, why your child doesn't correct a high blood sugar) can help you influence his behavior. If your child doesn't correct his blood sugar find out why: Is it because he fears he'll go too low? This kind of understanding does change behavior. Satin-Rapaport also agrees on the use of consequences to improve teens' responsibility and recommends rewarding responsible behavior with privileges. Positive reinforcement, such as letting your teen borrow the car, prompts desired behaviors and underscores how responsible behavior yields positive results. Like Solowiejczyk, who says he's the first to applaud teens when they're "doing the hard work," Satin-

Rapaport says you can empower your teen when you point out what he is doing well.

Partner with your teen

Helaine Ciporen, clinical social worker at the Department of Pediatric Endocrinology and Diabetes at Mount Sinai Hospital in New York City, says having a teenager with diabetes isn't just a teen issue; it's a family issue. Whether your teen got diabetes years ago or very recently, you can expect he will need additional support and structure as he goes through adolescence. "No matter when children were diagnosed, even if they've been living with diabetes since they were small, when they hit puberty you can feel like you're all starting from scratch," says Ciporen.

"Teenagers are in a rebellious stage of life and if they have diabetes, that will likely be the focus of their rebellion. All of a sudden kids who took care of themselves under their parents' supervision no longer want supervision. They may feel like *I just want to be like everyone else* and *I don't want to have this anymore.* They may act out, not take their insulin, forget their supplies and not even want their friends, who've known they've had diabetes for years, to know." But, Ciporen says, they still need supervision. Adolescents need to step up and take more responsibility, but parents shouldn't drop the reins entirely. It's a gradual transition from caretaker to partner.

Creating a supportive family structure

Operating as a family unit, with each member invested in the others' welfare, and laying down ground rules are critical to help your

---

Tip to Make You Tops

The first two diabetes interviews I did were with Marsha and her daughter Allison. Allison had just turned fourteen and had been diagnosed with diabetes when she was five. She'd been a model child taking care of her diabetes under her parent's supervision, but now Marsha and Allison were at odds trying to find a new path between mom letting go and Allison taking over. Last year Allison felt she should take more insulin than Marsha did. "I wouldn't let her because I was scared she'd go too low," said Marsha. That left Allison caught between wanting to do what she knew felt right and not wanting to offend her mother, until the doctor said to Marsha, "She's doing it right more than you, mom, just be quiet." "That was when I realized I had to start letting go," said Marsha. "Sometimes we're holding back and she's moving forward, sometimes the opposite, but Allison and I have formed a partnership. We have agreed to discuss things and work them out together."

---

teen take more accountability for his diabetes management. Solowiejczyk told me about a very sweet, very intelligent fifteen-year-old girl named Debbie whose health was suffering because she was tired of her mother's nagging about her poorly managed diabetes. Wanting to exert her power and independence, Debbie, who was doing well in every other area of her life, stopped checking her blood sugars regularly and often skipped her insulin injections. Solowiejczyk instructed Debbie's parents to handle these behaviors just as they would any other act of misbehavior.

Three weeks after Debbie's parents told her what their expectations were regarding her diabetes management and explained what consequences would be imposed if she didn't deliver, Debbie was doing six blood sugar checks a day, taking her shots before meals, and logging her blood sugars. The family meets weekly to discuss Debbie's results. They applaud excellent behavior, they mete out consequences as required (they took Debbie's laptop away from her for two days for two missed blood sugar checks), and the fights and tension have disappeared.

As a family, you should discuss and agree on

- What diabetes tasks your teenager will perform, such as doing his own blood sugar checks.
- Specific expectations. Solowiejczyk insists that a teen with type 1 diabetes must test at least four times a day and keep a record of all blood sugar tests.
- When and how often you'll meet to review results.
- The consequences for not following through and the rewards for completing tasks.

Leave judgment at the door

When interacting with your teen, encourage him to anticipate challenges, and facilitate ways to manage situations, for instance,

---

Tip to Make You Tops

"Children with Diabetes" is an online community that hosts an annual conference for families with diabetes. Parents attend educational and motivational workshops, and kids of all ages learn, play, and bond with other kids who have diabetes. Visit its Web site at www.childrenwithdiabetes.com.

LOOKING THROUGH THE LENS OF . . .
Joe Solowiejczyk, Family Therapist and Certified Diabetes Educator, and Wendy Satin-Rapaport, Licensed Clinical Psychologist

Five Ways to Take Care of Your Diabetes:

1. If your child has diabetes, do not lower expectations for yourself or your child to have a full, productive, happy, active life. Do give yourself time to make adjustments to the diagnosis.
2. Shape your child's behavior by focusing on improving his or her behaviors without making character judgments.
3. If you're the one with diabetes, be open to receiving help from loved ones and friends in managing it—you don't have to do it alone! For parents, try to get away occasionally to recharge.
4. Try not to "react" to numbers. They are only numbers, not measures of self-esteem or general health. Think through causes, patterns, and solutions, and abandon perfection as a goal.
5. All children need respectful supervision and collaboration, along with opportunities to become more empowered, until they are out of the house . . . and then some.

what teens may encounter if they go away to college. And always talk about other things, before diabetes, when your child first comes through the door.

Solowiejczyk, Satin-Rapaport, and Ciporen all say, don't judge your teen's actions. If your teen is hesitant or resistant to take on tasks, find out why. He may be afraid of your judgment, or he may be judging his own performance too critically. When reviewing blood sugars, listen to what your child has to say, empathize, and problem-solve. Use your teen's blood sugar numbers as information to reinforce what he is doing well and to determine where he may be having trouble.

When using rewards, be careful to reward the effort, not necessarily the outcome, because diabetes can't be managed perfectly. Try as hard as you might, you can't always create the outcome you want. And finally, Satin-Rapaport says, "You must parent your teen as though he didn't have diabetes."

MYTH #45

There's nothing good about having diabetes.

TRUTH: *Actually*, many people find diabetes a wake-up call to become healthier and an incentive to find greater meaning and purpose in life.

I have interviewed more than 120 people with diabetes, and many have told me diabetes has actually made them healthier. They have used it as motivation to change their diet—get rid of the junk food, watch their portions, and shed some pounds—and to *finally* commit to a more active lifestyle. Some, after their diagnosis, transformed from devoted couch potatoes into dedicated athletes, running marathons or biking. Others became just as fervently dedicated to a regular evening walk. Many have quit smoking and moderated their drinking, which lowered their blood pressure and cholesterol and increased their energy and vitality. I discovered that many people, after their diagnosis, illustrated the wisdom of the nineteenth-century English physician and philosopher Sir William Osler, who once said, "To live a long and healthy life, develop a chronic disease and take care of it."

Diabetes also serves frequently as a wake-up call for the entire family to engage in more healthful habits. Home-cooked meals replace frequent outings to McDonald's, and Sundays become family day in the park. Many people who got type 1 diabetes as children say that growing up with the disease made them more

Tom, a retired teacher, got type 1 diabetes at fifty and completely turned his life around, becoming a champion bicycler and a leader of several diabetes support groups. "I tell people I wouldn't wish diabetes on anyone, but I'm in the shape I'm in because of it," Tom told me. "Before, I was always eating pizza, drinking beer, or lying on the couch, and I'd still be doing that if I hadn't gotten diabetes. This morning I jumped on my bike and rode forty miles."

When Tom's doctor told him he had diabetes, Tom said, "Oh, no, you've got that wrong. Tell me what to do and I'll make this go away." Learning it doesn't work that way, Tom then said, "OK, tell me what I need to do and I'll do it." Shortly thereafter, Tom went to a DESA (Diabetes Exercise and Sports Association) conference where he met people "who put me to shame. Marathoners and Ironman competitors, ice climbers, and a gal who recently climbed a 23,000-foot mountain. I started out walking for exercise and then decided to do the Tour for the Cure bike ride and raise money for diabetes research. It was a struggle; I trained two months taking baby steps, but now I won't even get on the bike unless I'm going at least twenty-five miles.

"Diabetes pushed me to do things that have changed my life. If somehow tomorrow I woke up and diabetes was history, I'd still follow the same regimen and diet. A lot of people say they can't do what I've done or that it's easy for me, but I started biking when I was 55; it *wasn't* easy for me. Something's going to get me sooner or later, but it's not going to be diabetes. Whenever I go to my doctor, I tell him I'm the healthiest person he's going to see today."

mature, driven, and responsible; they're also more compassionate and sympathetic than they might have been otherwise.

Most people I spoke with also found something positive in their diabetes on a spiritual level. Of course, they would still welcome a cure this minute, and yet they appreciate that diabetes has opened their hearts and their eyes to blessings they already had and has prompted them to create an even richer and more satisfying life.

Finding greater purpose and meaning through diabetes

For many people, diabetes brought them to a crossroads where they began to more fully appreciate their family, friends, work, and community and found a desire to "give back." Making a difference and contributing to others tend to become deeper impulses as we age, yet many people find diabetes prompts these same desires. Many people I've spoken with have educated their fellow employees, spoken at schools, encouraged others, and shared their experience. Teaching others not only helps someone who is newly diagnosed, but also provides healing for the sharer. And even though managing diabetes can be challenging, people say it has also shown them their own strength, courage, resilience, and pride. A diabetes educator told me she often thinks of the adage, "Old age can make you bitter or make you better." She and I both think this is true of diabetes.

In the summer of 2008, a clever and moving video was developed by Nicholas Dewyer and Jane Lee, two young medical students with type 1 diabetes, as part of their coursework at the University of Michigan Medical School. We see onscreen a poem being revealed, line by line, and hear a voice narrating it. Then, midway through the video, the poem is scrolled backward line by line, and narrated in reverse—and this changes its entire meaning. Here's what the poem, "It Turned Everything Upside Down," says about living with diabetes:

It turned everything upside down
My identity and hope for the future
It stole the most important things from me
I would be lying to you if I said that
I have a great future ahead
That I could be promoted for my work
That my wife could sleep without fear
That my children could be safe and healthy
Following the initial shock, I recognize
I am happy
Only some of the time
Would I exchange my life for yours?
Amputations and vision loss are my inevitable future
Loneliness and shame are my chronic company and
I cannot and refuse to believe that
I am gaining strength and peace through this
The physical pain can be unbearable but
There are even more complications to come
I will not waste my time on how
There is hope that I can turn things around
I choose how I view my illness
Because whether I like it or not
I awake everyday into this reality
But while this direction may be the case for some
I experience exactly the opposite

Now read the poem in reverse, starting from the third-to-last line: "I awake everyday into this reality." See how completely the meaning changes from despair to hope and empowerment. If we think there is something to be gained from living with diabetes, we will be happier, and more successful, managing it.

My own litmus test of whether there's something good about having diabetes

On Valentine's Day 2008, I attended my local diabetes support group as the guest speaker to introduce a book I wrote and illustrated, *The ABCs of Loving Yourself with Diabetes.* I read from my book and then conducted an exercise with the group of twenty-six women there that evening. I asked everyone to say one positive thing diabetes has given them. Half the women mentioned appreciation or humility. One woman, who has diabetes-related eye disease, said she had more compassion for people with disabilities. Women who got diabetes young said it had helped them learn to be strong. Many women said diabetes has helped them eat healthier or get regular exercise or lose weight, and they were grateful for that. Some talked about the friendships they'd formed in the group. Many said they are helping family members with diabetes, which makes them feel worthy and valuable. For me, diabetes is a blessing in disguise: I have lost thirty pounds and kept them off for thirty years. I walk an hour almost every day, rain or shine, and am fit as a fiddle. I know how precious and fleeting time is, and I use mine to do things I really enjoy. I also see my strength reflected in my managing this illness every day. Diabetes has given me wonderful friends who share membership in this club and this work that I do now educating others, which provides me with a deep sense of purpose and satisfaction.

Carolyn, a remarkably youthful seventy-eight-year-old woman who has lived with type 2 diabetes for thirty-two years, says she feels better than ever. In the heyday of her career, Carolyn traveled to ninety-seven countries around the world as the national executive for a mission organization and loved it. "Now I give educational diabetes presentations in hospitals and churches to small groups of patients, and I get just as much pleasure," she said. "I'm an 'encourager' and I love that. I run through airports, get to the event site, and I'm on. I'm seventy-eight years old and I still have something to offer!"

Jan, an artist in her thirties, got diabetes at ten. She says, "Don't use diabetes to hold you back. If anything, use it to help you do something. My parents always had my best interest at heart, but they were afraid to let me go to sleep-away camp, and then away to college, and then to Israel when I went. I always wanted to do whatever anyone else could, and I've proven that I can. I really like who diabetes has made me; maybe I'd be the same without it, but I really don't think so."

Practical & Practices Myths

MYTH #46

Financial help for diabetes treatment, supplies, and education is not available to me.

TRUTH: *Actually,* Medicare, health insurance, and a number of pharmaceutical and government programs help defray the cost of supplies and education. Some even make them available at no charge to you.

Diabetes is an expensive disease to care for, and the truth is many people have to rely on either their employer's health insurance or Medicare to defray the costs. However, if you're uninsured or underinsured, there are actually many government and pharmaceutical assistance programs through which you can obtain necessary medicine, supplies, and education.

Medicare is available to people who are sixty-five years of age and older, to people who are under sixty-five and have certain disabilities, and to anyone with end-stage renal disease (permanent kidney failure requiring dialysis or a kidney transplant). Medicare covers the cost of glucose monitors, test strips, and lancets, along with educational training. Medicare also covers glaucoma screening and podiatry services, including special shoes and orthotics, or corrective shoe inserts, which can help reduce the chance of diabetic foot problems. If you need someone to help you through the maze of Medicare's offerings, you can call their general coverage hotline at 800-633-4227.

If you have health insurance, it's important to look at what your insurance does and doesn't cover. Some health insurance plans offer 100 percent coverage of your medicines and supplies (such as meters, lancets, test strips, and syringes); others make them available with a small co-pay; and some, unfortunately, do not cover these costs at all. A few years ago, my health care company merged with a medical durable supplies company, and after decades of co-pays I began receiving my syringes, test strips, and lancets free. A prescription drug plan lowers your costs for medicine, and using their mail-order pharmacy makes medicines even less expensive. Many drug plans' mail-order pharmacies provide a three-month supply of medications for a two-month co-pay.

Tip to Make You Tops

If your health insurance covers meters, it should also cover the test strips. If your health insurance has a durable medical equipment (DME) benefit, check there first for coverage of your supplies. It is usually more generous than a plan's pharmacy benefit.

Your physician may also be able to help you reduce some of the costs of diabetes care. He or she may be able to

1. Prescribe generic (rather than brand-name) supplies that cost less
2. Provide you free samples of medicines
3. Advise you of the critical times to test your blood sugar, so that you can use fewer test strips yet get the information you need to control your blood sugar

4. Direct you to community programs that provide medicines at lower costs

5. Write a letter on your behalf to an assistance program

Linda asks her provider whenever she sees him for insulin and usually receives four to six vials for free. "He has closets in his office full of medications that the pharmaceutical companies give him to give to patients." When she has a change in prescription, Linda brings any unopened and unused supplies back to her doctor's office and asks him to give them to someone who can use them.

The ADA provides financial assistance information

The American Diabetes Association's National Call Center handles 300,000 calls a year regarding financial assistance and offers guidance on confusing lists of benefits and co-pays. It can also offer advice to people looking for financial assistance programs or health insurance. You can call the National Call Center at 1-800-DIABETES (342-2383) or check their Web site at www.diabetes.org for information regarding

- How to find affordable health insurance
- Phone numbers for state insurance programs
- Saving money on supplies and medicines
- Resources such as Co-pay Relief, an organization that helps with co-pays, and other organizations offering financial assistance
- Financial assistance for people who have complications such as kidney disease, and prosthetics for amputees

- Supplies and free or low-cost health insurance for children under eighteen
- The names and addresses of diabetes education programs near you
- Educational classes for those unable to afford diabetes classes

---

Tip to Make You Tops

Ben Ortolaza, quality assurance specialist for the ADA, offers these ideas to lower your costs:

- Prescription assistance programs—Many local chains, such as Wal-Mart and Target, offer prescription assistance programs that make drugs available at greatly reduced cost.
- Generics—A nonbranded medicine may cost as much as 60 percent less than its branded version.
- The Roche Diagnostics patient assistance program—Offers free glucometers and medications to individuals who are unable to pay and are not eligible for public or private coverage. For information, call 1-866-441-4090.
- Split your pills in half—Ask your doctor to prescribe a dose twice what you need, and then split your pills in half. They'll cost the same and last twice as long.
- Buy the store-brand meter—Many brand names offer free meters, but the catch is that the test strips are expensive. You'll do better spending a little for the store-brand meter and a lot less for the test strips.
- Get as much, or as little, functionality as you need—The more bells and whistles on a meter, the more it will cost. If you need only the basics, don't buy an expensive meter.

Pharmaceutical companies help cut costs with patient assistance programs

Many pharmaceutical companies sell insulin and other diabetes medications through lower-cost patient assistance programs. These programs make prescribed medications attainable if you do not have health insurance and cannot otherwise afford them. Many of these programs, however, are available only through physicians, so if the cost of medicine and supplies is beyond your reach, it's important you talk to your health care provider. You generally need a letter or application from your doctor to enroll in one of these programs. The following pharmaceutical companies offer assistance programs. Be sure to call and see what information you may need to enroll.

Aventis	800-221-4025
Bayer Corporation	800-998-9180
Bristol-Myers Squibb	800-437-0994
Eli Lilly & Company	800-545-6962
Novo Nordisk	800-727-6500

Financial assistance information or programs

- *The Medicine Program* helps patients find and apply for free medicines supplied by some pharmaceutical companies. You can write to: The Medicine Program, P.O. Box 1089, Poplar Bluff, MO, 63902.
- *The Partnership for Prescription Assistance program* (PPA) offers information on prescription medicine assistance programs. To see whether you qualify, visit www.pparx.org or

call 1-888-477-2669. The PPA also connects people to free health clinics in their community.

- *The Pharmaceutical Research and Manufacturers of America* publishes the Directory of Prescription Drug Patient Assistance Programs. For a directory, write to Pharmaceutical Research and Manufacturers of America, 1100 Fifteenth Street, NW, Washington, DC, 20005.

- *The National Institute of Diabetes and Digestive and Kidney Diseases* (NIDDK) publishes a guide on financial resources called "Financial Help for Diabetes Care." For a copy, call 1-800-860-8747.

- *Together RX Program* offers savings of 25 to 40 percent on more than 300 prescription products. Visit www.together rxaccess.com or call 1-800-444-4106.

- *The Department of Health and Human Services* administers a program for hospital care if you are uninsured and provides free or reduced-cost medical services to people with lower incomes. For more information, visit www.hrsa.gov/hillburton/default.htm or call 1-800-638-0742.

- *The U.S. Department of Veterans Affairs* runs hospitals and clinics that will treat you for a modest cost even if you don't have a service-connected health problem. Visit www.va.gov or call 1-800-827-1000.

- *The Bureau of Primary Health Care* offers health care for people regardless of their insurance status or ability to pay. To find local health centers, visit www.bphc.hrsa.gov or call 1-800-400-2742.

- *Health and Human Services* helps people in need of medical care. Your local county or city government can provide further information.

Tip to Make You Tops

Two online companies can help you find out whether you qualify for a reduced-cost program or medication: www.freemedicine revolution.com and www.freedrugcard.us.

Self-management training and education

Diabetes education services are also covered by most health insurance plans, with your plan's approval and a referral from your physician. Your plan will probably indicate a number of classes or hours that it covers within a certain time period. Medicare, for instance, provides ten free hours of diabetes education per year and will cover two hours per year after the first year as follow-up.

If your plan does cover classes, check which ones. It may cover nutrition education but not walking programs, or it may cover only a particular organization's classes, such as those offered by the American Diabetes Association. Look also for free and low-cost diabetes education classes at your local library, YMCA, senior center, or hospital.

Many hospitals provide diabetes support groups that are free and often have a guest speaker who is a specialist in diabetes care. The American Diabetes Association, Taking Control of Your Diabetes (TCOYD), and "Divabetic: Makeover Your Diabetes" offer free one-day educational events across the country where you can attend workshops on various aspects of diabetes care; hear experts speak; talk individually with specialists; get your blood sugar, A1C, cholesterol, vision, and feet checked; see the latest diabetes tools and devices; and find the most current diabetes information.

#47

Once I begin using a bottle of insulin, it has to be refrigerated.

TRUTH: *Actually,* once you begin using a bottle of insulin, it can be kept at room temperature for up to twenty-eight days.

One of my earliest memories after my diagnosis is moving a half-sized refrigerator into my college dorm room to store my insulin. There, amid the two single beds, two wooden desks, and dayglow posters, was now a refrigerator and a constant reminder that my life was no longer carefree. The rule thirty years ago was that insulin had to be refrigerated while you were using it; but no longer. Although you should still store unused insulin in the fridge, once you've opened a bottle it can safely stay at room temperature, between 59°F and 86°F (15°C and 30°C), for up to twenty-eight days. This is because standard insulin preparations have preservatives in them that keep the insulin effective approximately this long. After twenty-eight days insulin loses potency, so it's best to discard it even if there's more in the vial.

If you use insulin from a bottle that's been opened more than twenty-eight days, you may begin to notice that your blood sugars are higher than usual for no apparent reason. Of course, the reason is that you're not getting a true dose from your weakened insulin. Because I don't use up a vial of insulin in four weeks, I store mine in the refrigerator while I'm using it; this helps extend its life a bit longer. To avoid any confusion, however, about whether your insulin isn't working at its maximum effectiveness or there's a medical reason why your blood sugars are high, it is best to discard your insulin after twenty-eight days.

Tip to Make You Tops

A handy way to tell how long you've been using your insulin is to mark your vial or insulin pen with the date when you start using it.

Don't let insulin get too hot or too cold

If insulin gets too hot or too cold, it can lose potency or become entirely ineffective. If you keep your insulin outside the refrigerator, don't place it anywhere it can get hot, such as on a windowsill, near the stove or a heater, or too close to a lamp. If you live in a hot or tropical climate, be aware that *your* room temperature may be above the recommended 86ºF (30ºC), especially during the summer. Never place insulin on the windshield of a car, where the beating sun can overheat it, or in the trunk of a car on a hot day. If you're traveling in a car without air conditioning on a very hot day, you might take a cool pack along for your insulin. Insulin should never freeze, however, because freezing causes the ingredients to "unmix" and renders the insulin useless.

I had a minor scare with my Lantus® on a hot day in July in Arizona. I flew in from New York to meet my book agent. Not being used to 102-degree-heat, or even to riding in cars, I put my suitcase, which contained my insulin, into the trunk of her car. It sat in there for three hours before we arrived at our destination.

When I took my case out of the trunk and reached for my insulin, it was hot to the touch. I knew it might not work.

We went right away to a drugstore to get another bottle of insulin, but without a current prescription issued in Arizona (this differs from state to state), I was out of luck. It was Saturday night, and knowing I couldn't reach my doctor, I called a friend who is a physician's assistant and was working in a pharmacy. She asked the pharmacist about my predicament, and he said I should check my Lantus®, normally a clear liquid, for clouding or crystals. If I saw any, my insulin might well have gone bad. If not, it was probably OK. Upon inspection, my Lantus® was clear as a bell, so I continued to use it but checked my blood sugar ten times the next day to be certain it was working.

I've since learned to be more careful with my insulin. Also, it's a good idea to check with your insulin's manufacturer and find out what they advise regarding insulin's potency after exposure to extreme temperatures.

Tip to Make You Tops

Frio bags keep insulin at a safe, cool temperature without refrigeration. They're available on many Web sites.

How to store insulin pens

Safe storage of insulin pens means following guidelines similar to those for storing vials of insulin. Store unused insulin pens in the refrigerator. When kept in the refrigerator, they are good until their expiration date. One diabetes educator advises her patients to store their pens on the refrigerator door so there's no chance they'll end up at the back of the fridge, a cold spot where they're at risk of freezing. Like bottles of insulin, insulin pens and insulin cartridges should never be allowed to freeze and should be kept away from direct heat and light.

Most manufacturers advise, however, that once you've begun using an insulin pen, it (unlike a vial of insulin) *should* be kept at room temperature. Cold insulin forms bubbles in the pen's insulin cartridge, which can prevent you from getting your full dose. Accordingly, manufacturers recommend that you take your pen out of the refrigerator one or two hours before the first time you use it. Because different manufacturers recommend using their pen for various numbers of days, check the package inserts, call the pen manufacturer, or visit the manufacturer's Web site so you will be familiar with the particular storage and usage guidelines for your pen.

I should never use a syringe, pen needle, or lancet more than once.

TRUTH: *Actually,* you can reuse all of these, as long as you follow certain guidelines.

The American Diabetes Association recommends that you use a new syringe, pen needle, or lancet for each injection, yet they say this is not an iron-clad rule. You can reuse these items if you take certain precautions. Diabetes educators agree with the ADA's recommendation, saying that in an ideal world it's best to use a needle (for brevity I will use "needle" to mean syringe, pen needle, and lancet) only once, but they also know that in the real world sometimes this just isn't possible. If you're traveling, for instance, you may not have packed enough needles, or it may be too costly for some patients to use a new needle each time.

Using a needle only once provides two basic benefits: (1) It helps keep the injection relatively painless and (2) it minimizes the risk of infection. That said, while I was discussing this issue with a diabetes educator who has diabetes herself, we both admitted we tend to reuse syringes until the injection begins to prick a little. In fact, I find that many people I know who take insulin injections do the same. However, I do follow the precautions the ADA recommends.

Needles can typically be used several times before the silicone coating dulls enough for injections to hurt or the needle gets

Tip to Make You Tops

The American Diabetes Association
guidelines if reusing needles

- Recap the syringe after you use it. If you have difficulty with manual dexterity, poor vision, or tremors and can't recap your syringe, use a new one each time you inject.
- Don't let the needle touch anything but your clean skin and your insulin bottle stopper. If it touches anything else, don't use it.
- Store the used syringe at room temperature.
- Use separate syringes for two different insulins, because there will always be a residual amount of insulin in the syringe.
- Do not reuse a needle that is bent or dull.
- Never share needles or use someone else's; germs can be spread, causing serious conditions such as HIV and hepatitis.
- Do not clean the needle with alcohol. This removes the coating that helps it glide smoothly into your skin.

chipped or damaged. However, needles are so thin and delicate today that I can vouch for the fact that they bend more easily than years ago. If a needle is bent and you reuse it, it can break off in your skin. Syringe manufacturers recommend that you use a syringe only once, largely because they cannot guarantee the needle will be sterile if you reuse it. If you have poor personal hygiene, are ill, have open wounds, or have a low resistance to infection, you definitely shouldn't reuse your syringes or you may risk infection.

Some diabetes educators recommend this general rule if you want to reuse your needles: Use the same needle for one day and start with a fresh one the next day. However, some educators caution specifically against reusing *pen needles,* because doing so can cause air to enter the insulin reservoir in the pen or the pen may leak when dosing. Both can cause inaccurate dosing.

Tip to Make You Tops

If you reuse syringes, periodically inspect the skin around your injection site to make sure there's no unusual redness or sign of infection.

How to dispose of used needles

The recommended way to dispose of needles is to use a Sharps container, a reusable, hard container made especially for this purpose. You can buy a Sharps container at most drug stores, including chains such as Wal-mart, and online for a few dollars. Some counties offer them free. Check with your local hospital about how and where to empty your Sharps container. I've adopted my friend Paula's needle disposal system. With my syringe capped, I snap the orange cap portion off the body of the syringe. I then store the capped portion in a coffee tin (a hard plastic container such as a laundry detergent bottle will work too) and throw the body of the syringe in the garbage. When the tin is full, I seal it with tape so that no one, such as an unsuspecting garbage collector, can open it accidentally and sustain an injury. Note: Check whether this disposal method is permitted in your local county. If not, you may be risking a hefty fine.

You can also use a tool called a needle clipper, available from Becton Dickinson, that clips the needle off your syringe and stores up to a two-year supply of needles right in the handy little device. Never flush needles down the toilet, and when traveling, bring your used needles home and dispose of them properly.

I can't bring syringes and other diabetes supplies aboard an airplane.

TRUTH: *Actually*, you can, and if you know the guidelines to follow, you won't be inconvenienced.

I travel a lot. I give diabetes presentations across the country and visit family across the Atlantic Ocean. Over the past few years, I've been in and out of airports in New York City, Bangor, Spokane, Sioux Falls, Orlando, Omaha, St. Louis, San Francisco, Sydney, Singapore, and Tokyo. Well, you get the idea. I've never once been stopped from carrying my syringes, test strips, insulin vials, insulin pens, meters, lancing devices, or lancets aboard an airplane or in my checked luggage. In fact, no security official has ever raised an eyebrow, not even an enthusiastic Welsh security officer who gave my cosmetics bag with syringes nestled at the bottom a vigorous hand-search in London. Maybe I've just been lucky, and not wanting to press my luck, I follow the U.S. Transportation Security Administration (TSA) guidelines for traveling with diabetes supplies.

Rules of the air: Flying with diabetes supplies

The official recommendation when being searched before boarding a plane is that passengers with diabetes should notify the U.S. Transportation Security Administration (TSA) Security Officer that they have diabetes and are carrying their supplies with them. If you're carrying syringes or wearing an insulin pump, they must be accompanied by insulin, and your insulin must be clearly identified by a pharmaceutical label. I carry in my wallet the side panel from my insulin box, which displays the insulin's name and my name; some people carry their insulin in its original box. If you're carrying lancets, they must be capped and accompanied by a glucose meter that has the manufacturer's name printed on it. Glucagon kits should be in their original containers with a pharmaceutical label. If you're traveling internationally, the same basic guidelines apply, and if you're traveling in a country where people are unfamiliar with an insulin pump, be sure to let the security official know it is a medical device.

In reality, most people I know say, as my friend Larry does, "I have never been questioned about carrying insulin, needles, or even ice and water in a bag to keep unopened insulin pens cool. I do have a letter from my doctor explaining that I am carrying insulin and needles to treat diabetes, but I have never been asked to show it." My experience is the same as Larry's, and I also carry in my wallet a note from my doctor on one of his prescription pad sheets, although it is not officially required.

The following diabetes-related supplies and equipment are allowed through the checkpoint once they have been screened.

- Insulin and insulin-loaded dispensing products (insulin pens, jet injectors, and preloaded syringes)
- Unlimited number of unused syringes
- Lancets, blood glucose meters, blood glucose meter test strips, alcohol swabs, and meter-testing solutions

- Insulin pump and insulin pump supplies (cleaning agents, batteries, plastic tubing, infusion kit, catheter, and needle)
- Glucagon emergency kit
- Urine ketone test strips
- Unlimited number of used syringes, when transported in Sharps disposal container or other, similar hard-surface container
- Sharps disposal containers or similar hard-surface disposal container for storing used syringes and test strips

---

Tip to Make You Tops

Airport X-ray machines won't hurt your glucose meter, insulin, or insulin pump. However, if you don't want to put your pump through the X-ray machine, the TSA allows you the option of a visual inspection. You must request it before the screening process begins. Also, be aware that an insulin pump may set off the walk-through metal detector. You can request a body pat-down instead. If you're being wanded, it's best to hold your pump in your outstretched hand and let the inspector wand around it.

You're permitted to bring prescription liquid medications such as insulin and other necessary liquids, such as juice, liquid nutrition, gels, and frozen liquids, in greater quantity than the three-ounce limitation on liquids. However, if you're carrying any of these liquids, other than insulin, in greater than three-ounce quantities, you must declare it to the Transportation Security Officer. I was stopped at the Sioux Falls airport when I had completely forgotten that I'd packed a five-ounce can of tomato juice in my luggage. I explained that I had diabetes and needed the juice in case of hypoglycemia. The officer called over his supervisor, who very pleasantly waved me through the hand search. Because not all TSA screeners are aware of the rules, it may help to carry these documents when traveling: *Travelers with Disabilities and Medical Conditions* and *Changes in Allowances for Persons with Disabilities at Airport Security Checkpoints.* They're posted on the TSA Web site at www.tsa.gov.

Here are some of my personal recommendations for flying with your diabetes supplies:

- Always take your diabetes supplies aboard with you, and never pack temperature-sensitive supplies in checked baggage, because temperatures in the cargo hold may harm them.
- Pack your supplies in duplicate and in separate pieces of luggage. Ask a friend to carry back-up supplies for you in his or her carry-on if necessary.
- Pack insulin vials between layers of clothing or in a protective sleeve or container. (Securitee blankets, available online, are softly padded inexpensive sleeves for your insulin.)
- Take more than enough supplies, perhaps an extra two weeks' worth, in case you lose them or don't return home on time.
- Have a current (within the last six months) prescription for your medicines.

If I wear an insulin pump, my diabetes is really "bad."

TRUTH: *Actually,* people who wear a pump do not have "worse" diabetes, and very often, they have better-controlled blood sugars.

Insulin pumps are miniature, computerized devices that deliver rapid- or short-acting insulin twenty-four hours a day through a few feet of tubing, where a thin, short plastic tube at the end is inserted just below the skin's surface. Insulin pumps are about the size of a pager, and they're typically worn on your waistband or in your pocket; many women actually wear them in their bra. People who use insulin pumps do so primarily for four reasons, and none of them is that their diabetes is more advanced than anyone else's. Most people use a pump because (1) It most closely mimics how the pancreas works, supplying a small continuous drip of insulin to cover metabolic functions, and, with the press of a few buttons, dispenses extra insulin to cover mealtime carbohydrates. (2) It makes correcting a high blood sugar painless and easy. (3) Its functionality makes it an extremely effective tool for keeping blood sugar in target range. (4) It affords wearers more freedom and flexibility with their mealtimes and exercise. The majority of pump users have type 1 diabetes, but anyone who uses insulin can use a pump.

As of this writing, there is one tubeless pump called the Om-niPod. The OmniPod consists of two separate components: an insulin reservoir in a shell-like pod and a wireless, handheld device that programs the pod. Some people dislike tubing because it can get caught on things. One young man told me his tubing frequently snagged on his doorknob when he was rushing out of his house to walk the dog. With the OmniPod's remote, you don't have to touch the pod to operate it, so you can wear it anywhere on your body. It's also lightweight. Some people don't like the OmniPod, however, because you can't take off the pod the way you can disconnect from a traditional pump for an hour at a time. You also have to replace the pod every three days, which means extra space is needed for storage and you'll be carrying quite a bit of equipment with you if you travel for any length of time.

Tip to Make You Tops

Many companies manufacture clothing specifically to hold insulin pumps. Pump Wear (www.pumpwearinc.com or 1-866-470-PUMP) specializes in children's clothing. Kangaroo Pump Pockets at www.mykpp.com specializes in children's and adults' needs.

Numerous studies show that most people who use a pump experience less hypoglycemia. Pumps enable you to better match your carbohydrates and exercise "moment-to-moment" because you can make immediate adjustments to your insulin delivery. Also, you actually need more insulin at certain times of day, such as in the morning when blood sugar is rising, and less at other times, such as during exercise, post-menses for many women, or if you have gastroparesis (slow stomach emptying). A pump enables you to pre-program greater and lesser amounts of insulin delivery at different times of day and night. If you don't use a pump and instead inject long-acting insulin once or twice a day, it's more difficult to accommodate these changing needs.

It should be said, however, that wearing a pump doesn't mean you'll automatically have perfect blood sugars. The pump has to be programmed and operated by its wearer, you, and using it requires that you calculate carbohydrates correctly, test your blood sugar frequently, and fine-tune your pump settings as needed.

Advantages of using an insulin pump

- Fewer needle sticks. You feel the prick of a needle only once every three days, when you insert the cannula (slender tube inserted into the body for insulin delivery), as opposed to multiple daily injections.
- Improved A1C. This is due to the pump's ability to deliver different amounts of insulin that more precisely match your needs.
- Connection to a continuous glucose monitor (CGM). The CGM is a little sensor device that gives a read-out of your blood sugar level every few minutes.
- Weight loss. By better matching your insulin to your activity, you can eliminate the need for extra carbohydrates.
- Knowing your insulin-on-board. Most pumps will tell you how much insulin you still have working from your last mealtime coverage.
- Carb-counting precision. Newer pumps include food databases with carb counts for hundreds of foods.

- Extended bolus. When dosing for foods that are digested slowly, such as beans, whole grains, dairy, and high fat-foods, a pump can deliver insulin in very small amounts over a prolonged period of time.

Tip to Make You Tops

All pump manufacturers offer pump training. They also offer a twenty-four-hour hotline and will gladly replace your pump if something goes wrong.

Disadvantages of using an insulin pump

- You must test your blood sugar at least four times a day. Even if using a CGM, today you still have to do finger sticks to confirm accuracy.
- There is the potential to gain weight, because it's easier to cover extra carbs with the push of a few buttons than by taking an injection.
- Pumps are expensive, particularly if not covered by insurance. They can cost up to $6,000.
- There is the possibility of malfunction, including a blockage or disrupted flow of insulin, which can cause high blood sugars.
- It can feel cumbersome to be attached to a device and tubing.
- The tubing can cause scarring or lesser insulin absorption after years of the cannula residing under the skin.
- You need to carry extra equipment, including insulin and syringes as a back-up.
- You need to be trained on the pump, to keep records, and to be extra diligent with your care.

Tip to Make You Tops

If you wear an insulin pump, always carry back-up supplies. My friend Ruth was in Denali, Alaska, when her pump battery nearly ran out. It was Sunday night, no store was open, and the nearby hospital didn't have the battery she needed. Ruth and her husband drove two and a half hours in a panic—because Ruth had no back-up insulin either—to Fairfax, where she got a battery just before her pump died.

When I give a diabetes presentation, people always ask me whether I wear an insulin pump, and the answer is "no." Primarily it's because I'm used to injections and don't mind them, I'm able to keep my A1C in the nondiabetic range through careful attention to my eating, exercise, and general health, and I don't want to have a piece of equipment attached to me. However, as I have told everyone, and will go on record as saying, when the insulin pump is closer to the size of a credit card, I will be the first one in line to get mine.

Acknowledgments

There's a reason why authors thank a long list of people, and now I know what it is. Simply, this book would not have been possible without the extraordinary generosity and collective knowledge and wisdom of my consulting experts. I am honored to have been a pupil at their feet. I thank Kathy Spain, who, without even being asked, became my well of support and practical knowledge, my clinical overseer, and my "Standards of Care" policewoman. I am also indebted to the following diabetes specialists, whose impressive titles are too long to list here: George W. Taylor, Richard K. Bernstein, Irl Hirsch, Seth Bernstein, Donna Rice, Kavita Pabby, Joy Pape, Susan Guzman, Helaine Ciporen, Gretchen Becker, and Joseph Stuto. I thank all my fellow peer-mentors and interns who shared their "lessons learned," as well as my editors, Matthew Lore, who set me on solid footing at the beginning, and Wendy Francis and Ashley St. Thomas, who brought this book home with a clear eye and welcome calm. Finally, my heartfelt thanks to my book agent, Claire Gerus, whose encouragement was invaluable throughout the writing of this book, and to my husband, Boudewijn, who has been and continues to be the wind beneath my sails.

Glossary

A1C: *See* Hemoglobin A1c.

Apidra: A rapid-acting insulin of relatively short duration (three to four hours).

Basal: The fasting state. Basal insulins are long-acting insulins that prevent blood sugar from rising while one is fasting.

Beta cells: Cells in the pancreas that produce and store insulin and amylin and secrete both into the blood stream.

Biofeedback: A technique to improve one's health by learning to control certain internal bodily processes that normally occur involuntarily, such as heart rate, blood pressure, muscle tension, and skin temperature.

Body mass index (BMI): A number calculated from a person's weight and height that provides an indicator of body fatness and is used to determine potential health risks.

Bolus: The administration of insulin at mealtimes to cover carbohydrates and keep blood sugar levels within normal range.

Cannula: A flexible plastic tube attached to an insulin pump with a small needle at the end that is inserted through the skin into the top layer of fatty tissue to deliver a constant insulin drip.

Carbohydrate: One of the major food groups, including simple sugars and more complex starches. Carbohydrates are the body's main energy source and are the nutrients that most raise blood sugar. Also referred to as "carb."

Celiac disease: A digestive disease that damages the small intestine and interferes with absorption of nutrients from food. People who have celiac disease cannot tolerate gluten, a protein in wheat, rye, and barley.

Complex carbohydrate: Made from longer, more complex chains of sugar. These are digested more slowly, and raise blood sugar less rapidly, than simple carbohydrates.

Diabetes: *See* type 1 diabetes; type 1.5 diabetes; type 2 diabetes; gestational diabetes.

Estimated average glucose (eAG): A mathematical translation of the A1C value into the same unit that glucometers display (mg/dl in the United States and mmol/l outside of the United States).

Fasting blood glucose: The blood sugar value before the first meal of the day.

Fat: A source of calories and energy in food that is high in calories. Fat does not directly raise blood sugar and can slow the rise of blood sugar when consumed with carbohydrate.

Foot ulcer: An open sore on the foot that can either be a shallow crater involving only the surface skin or extend through the full thickness of the skin, involving tendons, bones, and other deep structures. Foot ulcers are the most common cause of lower extremity amputation.

Gastroparesis: A neuropathy that is caused by prolonged high blood sugar and in which the stomach is slow to empty its contents. This causes blood sugar after meals to be unpredictable. Also called delayed stomach emptying,

Gestational diabetes: A condition in which women exhibit high blood glucose levels during pregnancy. A diagnosis of gestational diabetes is a risk marker for developing type 2 diabetes.

Glaucoma: A group of eye diseases associated with a buildup of internal eye pressure that can damage the eye's optic nerve and result in vision loss and blindness.

Glucagon: A hormone that is produced by the pancreas and causes blood sugar to rise.

Glucagon emergency kit: A small kit available at pharmacies and consisting of an injectable that releases the body's stored glucose in order to raise blood sugar quickly when a patient is experiencing severe hypoglycemia and is unable to ingest carbohydrate.

Glucose: Sugar in the blood stream; also, a building block of most carbohydrates.

Glycogen: A starchy substance that is formed from glucose and is made by, and stored in, the liver and muscles. It can rapidly be converted into glucose.

Hashimoto's disease: An autoimmune disorder resulting from the immune system attacking the thyroid gland, upsetting the balance of chemical reactions in the body. The inflammation caused by Hashimoto's disease most often leads to an underactive thyroid gland (hypothyroidism).

HDL: High-density lipoprotein, a particle that is found in the blood and is believed to offer protection from coronary artery disease. Also known as "good cholesterol."

Hemoglobin A1c: A blood value that reflects average blood glucose for the past two to three months. The Hemoglobin A1c (A1C) test measures what percentage of a person's hemoglobin—a protein in red blood cells that carries oxygen—is bonded with sugar (glycated).

Hyperglycemia: Abnormally high blood sugar.

Hypertension: High blood pressure.

Hypoglycemia: Abnormally low blood sugar, defined as blood sugar below 70 mg/dl (3.9 mmol/l).

Hypoglycemic unawareness: Inability to experience or perceive the physical symptoms of abnormally low blood sugar.

Insulin: A hormone that is produced by the beta cells in the pancreas and facilitates the entry of glucose into most cells in the body.

Insulin resistance: Reduced sensitivity to insulin's effect on blood sugar, either because the pancreas does not produce enough insulin or because the body does not use insulin effectively. Associated with obesity.

Ketoacidosis: An acute, life-threatening condition that is caused by hyperglycemia and dehydration and that affects people with type 1 diabetes. Ketone production and acidification of the blood causes Ketoacidosis.

Ketone: Fat deposits produced when fatty acids are broken down for energy.

Latent autoimmune diabetes in adults (LADA): A genetically linked, hereditary autoimmune disorder that causes the body to mistake the pancreas as foreign and to respond by attacking and destroying the insulin-producing beta islet cells of the pancreas.

LDL: Low-density lipoprotein, a particle in the blood that deposits cholesterol and triglycerides in arterial walls. Elevated LDL is a risk factor for coronary artery disease and peripheral vascular disease.

Lipid: A fat or fat-like substance found in the blood, such as cholesterol.

Macrovascular: Related to large blood vessels in the body.

mg/dl: Milligrams per deciliter, the unit in which blood sugar is measured in the United States.

Microvascular: Related to small blood vessels in the body.

mmol/l: Millimoles per liter, the unit in which blood sugar is measured outside of the United States (1 mmol/l = 18 mg/dl).

Nephropathy: A complication of diabetes due to elevated blood glucose that causes kidney damage and disease.

Neuropathy: A complication of diabetes due to elevated blood glucose that causes nerve damage.

Oral glucose tolerance test: Measures the body's ability to use glucose, the body's main source of energy. Usually performed in the morning after several hours' fast, this test consists of drinking a glucose-rich solution and drawing blood two hours afterward to measure glucose levels.

Oral medication: Pills used to lower blood glucose in type 2 diabetes.

Pancreas: An abdominal organ that manufactures and secretes into the blood stream insulin, glucagon, and other hormones and enzymes.

Peripheral neuropathy: A complication of diabetes that causes nerve damage resulting in pain, typically described as tingling or burning and numbness in the hands and feet. Loss of sensation is often compared to the feeling of wearing a thin stocking or glove.

Postprandial: After a meal; typically refers to a blood test taken two hours after beginning a meal.

Pre-diabetes: An abnormal state of high glucose that raises a person's risk of developing type 2 diabetes, heart disease, and stroke. Once referred to as "borderline" diabetes.

Retinopathy: Injury to the retina, the light-sensing surface in the back of the eye. Usually caused by chronically high blood sugars.

Simple carbohydrate: A carbohydrate that can be rapidly converted to glucose by the digestive process. Also called simple sugar.

Sulfonylureas: A class of oral glucose-lowering medications that stimulate beta cells to produce more insulin.

Triglycerides: Fats found in blood and fatty tissues. Elevated triglycerides, which are often the result of elevated blood sugar, are a risk factor for vascular disease.

Type 1 diabetes: One of the major types of diabetes, characterized by a total or near total loss of the capacity to produce insulin. Affects children in larger numbers than adults. Previously called juvenile diabetes.

Type 1.5 diabetes: A form of diabetes, sometimes called "double diabetes," in which a person has aspects of both type 1 and type 2 diabetes.

Type 2 diabetes: The most common type of diabetes, characterized by partial loss of insulin-producing capability and/or resistance to the effect of insulin. Usually appearing after age forty-five and commonly associated with overweight, obesity, and being sedentary. Previously called adult-onset diabetes.

Vascular: Related to blood vessels.

References

MYTH 1

"Diabetes and the American Diabetes Association," a fact sheet from the ADA.

"National Diabetes Fact Sheet, 2007." Department of Health and Human Services, Centers for Disease Control and Prevention. http://www.cdc.gov/diabetes/pubs/pdf/ndfs_2007.pdf.

MYTH 2

"Thin People Can Be Fat on the Inside." 2007. Associated Press. http://www.msnbc.msn.com/id/18594089/.

O'Connell, Jeff. "Even a Thin Person Can Get Diabetes." 2008. *Men's Health*. msnbc.com. http://www.msnbc.msn.com/id/24716880/.

MYTH 3

"Pre-Diabetes." 2007. WebMD. http://diabetes.webmd.com/guide/pre-diabetes.

"Fasting Plasma Glucose below 100 mg/dl and Risk of Type 2 Diabetes Diagnosis." 2008. Diabetes In Control.com. http://www.diabetesincontrol.com/results.php?storyarticle=5881.

"15 percent Increase in Diabetes in 2 Years." 2008. Diabetes In Control.com. http://www.diabetesincontrol.com/results.php?storyarticle=5882.

"A New Approach to Treating Type 2?" 2008. American Diabetes Association. http://americandiabetesnow.typepad.com/american_diabetes_associa/2008/06/a-new-approach.html.

"As Diabetes Becomes a Growing Concern, a Consensus Is Developing for Assertive Treatment of Pre-Diabetes." 2008. *Diabetes Health*. http://www.diabeteshealth.com/read/2008/09/04/5889.html.

"Pre-Diabetes." American Diabetes Association. http://www.diabetes.org/pre-diabetes.jsp.

"Diabetes Prevention Program." 2008. National Diabetes Information Clear-inghouse. http://diabetes.niddk.nih.gov/dm/pubs/preventionprogram/.

"National Diabetes Fact Sheet." 2005. National Center for Chronic Disease Prevention and Health. http://www.cdc.gov/diabetes/pubs/general.htm.

"Rapid, Non-Invasive Detection of Diabetes-Induced Retinal Metabolic Stress." 2008. *Archives of Ophthalmology* 126 (7): 934–938.

MYTH 4

Rodriguez, LuAnn. "Still Healthy after 54 Years Living with Type 1." 2008. http://www.diabeteshealth.com/read/2008/05/08/5744/still-healthy-after-54-years-living-with-type-1/

Colberg, Sheri, PhD, and Steven Edelman, MD. *50 Secrets of the Longest Living People with Diabetes* (New York: Marlowe, 2007).

Pérez-Peña, Richard. "Diabetic Brothers Beat Odds with Grit and Luck." *New York Times, February 5, 2006.*

MYTH 5

"UK Prospective Diabetes Study." *The Diabetes Monitor.* http://www.diabetes-monitor.com/d03.htm.

"Complications of Diabetes in the United States." American Diabetes Association. http://www.diabetes.org/diabetes-statistics/complications.jsp.

"Uric Acid Provides Early Clues to Diabetic Kidney Disease." 2008. *Clinical Journal of the American Society of Nephrology.* Diabetes In Control.com. http://www.diabetesincontrol.com/results.php?storyarticle=5626.

"When Does Diabetes Begin, and How Do We Know It?" 1997. *Clinical Diabetes.* Alan J. Garber, MD, PhD, Editor. http://journal.diabetes.org/clinicaldiabetes/v15n4J-A97/editoria.htm.

Manning, Anita. "Diabetes 'Revolution' Is Cutting Both Ways." 2007. *USA TODAY.* http://www.usatoday.com/news/health/2007-11-11-diabetes-cover_N.htm.

"Prevalence of Diabetes and Impaired Fasting Glucose in Adults—United States, 1999–2000." 2003. Department of Health and Human Services, Centers for Disease Control and Prevention. http://www.cdc.gov/mmwr/preview/mmwrhtml/mm5235a1.htm.

MYTH 6

Spain, Kathy, RN, BSN, CDE. "Do I Have Type 1 Diabetes or Type 2 Diabetes?" 2008. *Diabetes Explorer Magazine* 3 (1): 12–14.

"Children and Type 2 Diabetes." Canadian Diabetes Association. http://www .diabetes.ca/Section_about/children-type2-diabetes.asp.

Park, Alice. "Overweight Children: Living Large." 2008. *Time Magazine.* http:// www.time.com/time/magazine/article/0,9171,1813962,00.html.

Tennen, Melissa. "Adults Can Get 'Child' Diabetes." Health A to Z. http:// www.healthatoz.com/healthatoz/Atoz/common/standard/transform.jsp?requestURI=/healthatoz/Atoz/dc/caz/diab/dia1/alert08052003.jsp.

Parker-Pope, Tara. "Hint of Hope as Child Obesity Rate Hits Plateau." 2008. *New York Times.* http://www.nytimes.com/2008/05/28/health/research/ 28obesity.html.

MYTH 7

Satin-Rapaport, Wendy, Rebecca Taylor Cohen, and Matthew C. Riddle, MD. "Diabetes Through the Life Span: Psychological Ramifications for Patients and Professionals." 2000. *Diabetes Spectrum* 13 (4): 201.

MYTH 8

"Reduction in the Incidence of Type 2 Diabetes with Lifestyle Intervention or Metformin." *The New England Journal of Medicine* 346 (6): 60–64.

Hu, Frank B., MD, JoAnn E. Manson, MD, Meir J. Stampfer, MD, Graham Colditz, MD, Simin Liu, MD, Caren G. Solomon, MD, and Walter C. Willett, MD. "Diet, Lifestyle, and the Risk of Type 2 Diabetes Mellitus in Women." 2001. *The New England Journal of Medicine.*

MYTH 9

McCarren, Marie. "Sugar and Diabetes: The Myth That Won't Die." 2008. Woodacre, California. *Diabetes Health.* http://www.diabeteshealth.com/ read/2008/06/26/5806.html.

Keith, Sharon. "How to Eat and Live Healthier with Complex Carbohydrates and Fiber." eHow. http://www.ehow.com/how_2208950_live-healthier-complex-carbohydrates-fiber.html.

MYTH 10

"Implications of the United Kingdom Prospective Diabetes Study." 2003. *Diabetes Care* 26: S28–S32.

"The Diabetes Control and Complications Trial and Follow-Up Study." 2008. National Diabetes Information Clearinghouse. http://diabetes.niddk.nih.gov/dm/pubs/control/.

Parker-Pope, Tara. "Diabetes: Underrated, Insidious and Deadly." 2008. *New York Times.* http://www.nytimes.com/2008/07/01/health/01well.html.

MYTH 11

"Foot Care and Diabetes." 2005. The American College of Foot & Ankle Orthopedics & Medicine. http://www.acfaom.org/diabetes.shtml.

Manning, Anita. "Diabetes 'Revolution' Is Cutting Both Ways." 2007.

MYTH 13

Park, Alice. "The Kiddie Cholesterol Debate." 2008. *Time Magazine.* http://www.time.com/time/health/article/0,8599,1821153,00.html.

Park, Alice. "Overweight Children: Living Large." 2008. *Time Magazine.* http://www.time.com/time/magazine/article/0,9171,1813962,00.html.

Adams, Amy, MS. "Preventing Type 1 Diabetes." 2000. Genetic Health. http://www.genetichealth.com/DBTS_Prevention_for_Type_1_Diabetes.shtml.

Walsh, Bryan. "It's Not Just Genetics." 2008. *Time Magazine.* http://www.time.com/time/magazine/article/0,9171,1813984–1,00.html.

Kaufman, Francine R., MD. *Diabesity—The Obesity-Diabetes Epidemic That Threatens America and What We Must Do to Stop It* (New York: Bantam Books, 2005).

MYTH 14

Pape, Joy, RN, BSN, CDE, WOCN, FCNC. "I Don't Want to Wear Ugly Shoes! Especially During the Holidays!" dLife: For Your Diabetes Life! http://www.dlife.com/dLife/do/ShowContent/inspiration_expert_advice/expert_columns/pape_dec_2005.html.

MYTH 15

"Controlling Medication-Related Weight Gain." 2006. Johns Hopkins Health Alert. http://www.johnshopkinshealthalerts.com/alerts/diabetes/JohnsHopkins DiabetesHealthAlert_416–1.html.

Wartburg, Linda von. "Symlin Promising as Weight Loss Drug." 2007. DiabetesHealth. http://www.diabeteshealth.com/read/2007/10/12/5485.html.

Dairman, Tara. "Symlin May Help Obese People Lose Weight." 2007. Diabetes Self-Management. http://www.diabetesselfmanagement.com/blog/Tara_Dairman/Symlin_May_Help_Obese_People_Lose_Weight.

MYTH 16

"What Is Type 1 Diabetes?" 2006. Childrenwithdiabetes.com. http://www.childrenwithdiabetes.com/d_0n_100.htm.

MYTH 17

"Type 2 Diabetes May Be Caused by Intestinal Dysfunction; Research in Diabetes Surgery Offers Clues to Origins of the Disease" (New York: Weill Cornell Medical College, 2008). http://news.med.cornell.edu/wcmc/wcmc_2008/03_05_08.shtml.

Bernstein, Richard. *Dr. Bernstein's Diabetes Solution, a Complete Guide to Achieving Normal Blood Sugars* (Boston: Little, Brown, 1997).

Dotinga, Randy. "Gastric Lap-Band Surgery Can Send Diabetes into Remission." 2008. HealthDay News, ScoutNews, LLC, Medicine Net.

MYTH 18

"Rubino, Francesco." *Physician's Home Page.* Weill Cornell Medical College. http://www.cornellphysicians.com/frrubino/index.html.

"The Bypass Effect on Diabetes, Cancer." 2008. CBS News, *60 Minutes.* http://www.cbsnews.com/stories/2008/04/17/60minutes/main4023451.shtml.

"Innovative Diabetes Surgery Program Debuts." 2008. *The Scope* 1: 4.

"ADA: Glycemic Control Markedly Improved with Duodenal-Jejunal Sleeve." 2008. Diabetes In Control.com. http://www.diabetesincontrol.com/results.php?storyarticle=5844.

"A New Approach to Treating Type 2?" 2008. American Diabetes Association. http://americandiabetesnow.typepad.com/american_diabetes_associa/2008/06/a-new-approach.html.

"Type 2 Diabetes May Be Caused by Intestinal Dysfunction; Research in Diabetes Surgery Offers Clues to Origins of the Disease" (New York: *Weill Cornell Medical College, 2008*).

Pollack, Andrew. "Betting an Estate on Inhaled Insulin." 2007. *New York Times.* http://www.nytimes.com/2007/11/16/business/16mannkind.html?pagewanted=all.

Manning, Anita. "Diabetes 'Revolution' Is Cutting Both Ways." 2007.

Park, Alice. "Gastric Bypass Surgery Less Helpful for Diabetics." 2008. Time Inc. http://www.time.com/time/health/article/0,8599,1841440,00.html?xid=feed-cnn-topics.

Terry, Jaron. "Islet Cell Transplant: Is This the Cure for Type 1 Diabetes?" 2007. The Ohio State University Medical Center. http://medicalcenter.osu.edu/patientcare/healthcare_services/publications/?ID=2246.

Ewers, Justin. "Medications: Edging Closer to a Cure." 2007. *Scientific American.* http://www.sciam.com/article.cfm?id=medications-edging-closer-to-cure.

Ewers, Justin. "Managing Diabetes." *Scientific American Body Magazine* (2008): 46–54.

Spain, Kathy, BSN, CDE, RN. "Bariatric Surgery: Can It Cure Type 2 Diabetes?" 2007. *Diabetes Explorer Magazine* 2 (2): 33–36.

MYTH 19

Diabetes Self-Management Answer Book, 501 Tips and Secrets to Keep You Healthy, ed. James Hazlett (New York: Diabetes Self-Management Books, 2004).

MYTH 20

"Treating High Blood Pressure in People with Diabetes." American Diabetes Association. http://www.diabetes.org/type-1-diabetes/well-being/treating-high-bp.jsp.

"High Blood Sugar Levels a Risk Factor for Heart Disease." 2005. *Science Daily.* http://www.sciencedaily.com/releases/2005/09/050914105425.htm.

Manzella, Debra, RN. "Don't Forget Your Diabetes Check-Ups." 2007. About.com. http://diabetes.about.com/od/doctorsandspecialists/a/diabetescheckup.htm.

Staff, Mayo Clinic. 2007. *Diagnostic Tests.* MayoClinic.com. http://www .mayoclinic.com/health/diabetes-lab-tests/DA00104.

MYTH 21

Walsh, John, PA, CDE, and Ruth Roberts, MA. "Humalog® and Novolog® Insulins." Diabetes Mall. http://www.diabetesnet.com/diabetes_treatments/ insulin_humalog.php.

MYTH 22

"New Non-Invasive Technology Can View and Track Cells." 2008. Diabetes In Control.com. http://www.diabetesincontrol.com/results.php?storyarticle= 6027.

"Stem-Cell Breakthrough Brings Diabetes Cure Nearer." 2008. Diabetes In Control.com. http://www.diabetesincontrol.com/results.php?storyarticle= 6157.

Trecroci, Daniel. "Planting the Seeds for an Artificial Pancreas." 2000. Diabetes Health. http://www.diabeteshealth.com/read/2000/09/01/2001.html.

Spain, Kathy, RN, BSN, CDE. "An Alternative to Insulin Injections — Oral Insulin." 2008. *Diabetes Explorer* 3 (1): 70–71.

"Smart Insulin Nanostructures Pass Feasibility Test, Study Reports." 2007. ScienceDaily. http://www.sciencedaily.com/releases/2007/09/07092016 0236.htm.

Fox, Maggie. "Artificial Pancreas Just Years Away, Experts Agree." 2008. Reuters. http://www.reuters.com/article/healthNews/idUSN26405959200 80726?pageNumber=1&virtualBrandChannel=0.

MYTH 23

"Type 1 Diabetes and Pregnancy: Preparing for Pregnancy." JDRF. http:// www.jdrf.org/index.cfm?fuseaction=home.viewPage&page_id=EFEF9969 -1279-D3DC-F96062D5E5283E48.

"Preconception Risk Reduction." 2007. March of Dimes. http://www.march ofdimes.com/professionals/19695_1197.asp.

Kitzmiller, John L., MD, MS. "Managing Preexisting Diabetes for Pregnancy." 2008. *Diabetes Care* 31: 1060–1079.

MYTH 24

Tennen, Melissa. "Stress Can Aggravate Diabetes." 2007. Health A to Z. http://www.healthatoz.com/healthatoz/Atoz/common/standard/transform.jsp?requestURI=/healthatoz/Atoz/dc/caz/diab/dia2/alert03302004.jsp.

Surwit, Richard. *The Mind-Body Diabetes Revolution* (New York: Marlowe, 2004).

MYTH 26

Tsang, Gloria, RD. "High Blood Pressure Diet: The Dash Diet." 2006. Health-Castle.com. http://www.healthcastle.com/high-blood-pressure-diet.shtml.

Scritchfield, Rebecca. "Approaches to Mindful Eating." 2008. http://rebecca scritchfield.wordpress.com/2008/05/14/approaches-to-mindful-eating/.

MYTH 28

Weiner, Susan, RD, MS, CDE, CDN. "Healthy Swaps." 2008. dLife: For Your Diabetes Life! http://www.dlife.com/dLife/do/ShowContent/food_and_nutrition/menu_planning/healthy_swaps.html.

MYTH 32

Diabetes Self-Management Answer Book, 501 Tips and Secrets to Keep You Healthy, ed. James Hazlett (New York: Diabetes Self-Management Books, 2004).

Brown, Anthony J., MD. "Findings Show How Alcohol Lowers Blood Sugar." (New York: Reuters Health, 2008).

MYTH 33

"Kaiser Permanente Study Finds Keeping a Food Diary Doubles Diet Weight Loss." 2008. Kaiser Permanente. http://www.eurekalert.org/pub_releases/2008-07/kpdo-kps062308.php.

Nichols, Gregory A., PhD. "Weight Loss After Diabetes Diagnosis Improves Outcomes." 2008. Diabetes In Control.com. http://www.diabetesincontrol.com/results.php?storyarticle=6016.

Fuhrman, Joel, MD. *Eat to Live: The Revolutionary Formula for Fast and Sustained Weight Loss* (New York: Little, Brown, 2005).

MYTH 34

"Benefits of Exercise: Exercise and Diabetes: How Much Is Enough? Exercising with Limited Mobility." 2008. About, Inc., A part of The New York Times Company. http://diabetes.about.com/od/benefitsofexercise/Benefits_of_Exercise.htm

"Working Out, the Buddy System." 2008. *Health Monitor.* http://www.healthmonitor.com/featured/diabetes/working-out-buddy-system.html.

MYTH 35

"Diabetic Foot." 2001. American Academy of Orthopaedic Surgeons, Co-Developed by the American Orthopaedic Foot and Ankle Society. http://orthoinfo.aaos.org/topic.cfm?topic=A00148.

MYTH 36

"Diabetic Retinopathy." 2008. National Eye Institute. http://www.nei.nih.gov/health/diabetic/retinopathy.asp. [Adapted from Don't Lose Sight of Diabetic Eye Disease (NIH Publication No. 04–3252) and Diabetic Retinopathy: What You Should Know (NIH Publication No. 03–2171).]

Diabetes Self-Management Answer Book, 501 Tips and Secrets to Keep You Healthy, ed. James Hazlett (New York: Diabetes Self-Management Books, 2004).

Gordon, Serena. "Diabetes Seems to Heighten Glaucoma Risk." 2008. Medicine Net.com. http://www.medicinenet.com/script/main/art.asp?articlekey=89226.

"What Is Neovascular Glaucoma?" Glaucoma Associates of Texas. http://www.glaucomaassociates.com/neovascular-glaucoma.html.

MYTH 37

"Standards of Medical Care." 2008. *Diabetes Care* 31, Suppl. 1.

MYTH 38

"Erectile Dysfunction and Diabetes: Take Control Today." 2007. MayoClinic.com. http://www.mayoclinic.com/health/erectile-dysfunction/DA00045.

Manzella, Debra, RN. "Diabetes and Erectile Dysfunction." 2008. About.com. http://diabetes.about.com/od/preventingcomplications/qt/erectiledysfunc.htm.

Diabetes Self-Management Answer Book, 501 Tips and Secrets to Keep You Healthy, ed. James Hazlett (New York: Diabetes Self-Management Books, 2004).

MYTH 39

Diabetes Self-Management Answer Book, 501 Tips and Secrets to Keep You Healthy, ed. James Hazlett (New York: Diabetes Self-Management Books, 2004).

Rice, Birgitta, MS, RPh, CHES. "Pain in Your Feet? Try These Proven Techniques for Soothing Them." 2008. Diabetes Health. http://www.diabetes health.com/read/2008/01/31/5636.html.

Copeland, Lisa. "Antioxidant Alpha Lipoic Acid (ALA) Significantly Improves Symptoms of Diabetic Neuropathy." 2003. MayoClinic.com. http://www .newmayoclinicdiet.com/news2003-rst/1733.html.

"Antioxidant Alpha Lipoic Acid (ALA) Significantly Improves Symptoms of Diabetic Neuropathy." 2003. Science Blog Mayo Clinic. http://www.science blog.com/community/older/2003/F/20033816.html.

MYTH 40

"Periodontitis Associated with Development of Type 2 Diabetes and Its Complications." 2008. Diabetes In Control.com. http://www.diabetesincontrol .com/results.php?storyarticle=5828.

Diabetes Self-Management Answer Book, 501 Tips and Secrets to Keep You Healthy, ed. James Hazlett (New York: Diabetes Self-Management Books, 2004).

Bernstein, Richard, MD, FACE, FACN, CWS, FACCWS. *Dr Bernstein's Diabetes Solution 2007 Revised and Updated! A Complete Guide to Achieving Normal Blood Sugars* (Boston, Little, Brown, 2007).

MYTH 41

Polonsky, William, PhD. *"The Emotional Side of Diabetes, 10 Things You Need to Know"* (San Diego, CA: Behavioral Diabetes Institute, 2007).

MYTH 42

Satin-Rapaport, Wendy, LCSW, PsyD; Rebecca Taylor Cohen, MA; and Matthew C. Riddle, MD. "Diabetes Through the Life Span: Psychological Ramifications for Patients and Professionals." *Diabetes Spectrum* 13 (4): 201.

MYTH 43

Tenderich, Amy. "Top 10 Patient Gripes." 2008. Diabetes Health. http://www
.diabeteshealth.com/read/2008/09/22/4892.html.

MYTH 44

Solowiejczyk, Joe, RN, MSW. "The Family Approach to Diabetes Management: Theory into Practice Toward the Development of a New Paradigm."
2004. *Diabetes Spectrum*. American Diabetes Association. http://spectrum
.diabetesjournals.org/cgi/content/abstract/17/1/31.

MYTH 45

Lagergren, Eric. "'It Turned Everything Upside Down.'" 2008. *Diabetes Self-
Management*. http://www.diabetesselfmanagement.com/blog/Eric_Lagergren/
It_Turned_Everything_Upside_Down.

MYTH 46

"Preventive Services, Diabetes Screening, Supplies, and Self-Management Training." 2008. HHS.gov. http://www.medicare.gov/Health/Diabetes.asp.
"Financial Help for Diabetes Care." 2004. National Diabetes Information
Clearinghouse. http://diabetes.niddk.nih.gov/dm/pubs/financialhelp/.
Scheiner, Gary, MS, CDE. "Finding Financial Relief; Programs Are Available
to Help Offset the Cost of Diabetes Care." 2007. BD Diabetes.com.
http://www.bddiabetes.com/us/pdf/bd_update_45.pdf.
Spain, Kathy, RN, BSN, CDE. "Answerbook." 2007. *Diabetes Explorer Magazine* 2 (3): 8–10.

MYTH 47

"How to Store Insulin." Diabetes Mall. http://www.diabetesnet.com/diabetes
_treatments/insulin_basics.php.
McKinney, Christine, MS, RD, CDE. "Insulin Pens: Are You Using Yours Correctly?" 2007. Johns Hopkins University. http://health.yahoo.com/experts/
diabetesmckinney/30/insulin-pens-are-you-using-yours-correctly.

MYTH 48

American Diabetes Association Complete Guide to Diabetes, 4th ed. (New York: Bantam Books, 2006).

MYTH 49

"Hidden Disabilities: Travelers with Disabilities and Medical Conditions." Transportation Security Administration. http://www.tsa.gov/travelers/airtravel/specialneeds/editorial_1374.shtm.

MYTH 50

"About Omnipod Faqs." 2008. Insulet Corporation. http://www.myomnipod.com/products/section/226/.

"Insulin Pumps." ADA. http://www.diabetes.org/type-1-diabetes/insulin-pumps.jsp.

Index